MW00352756

PLANTED PERFORMANCE

EASY PLANT-BASED RECIPES, MEAL PLANS, AND NUTRITION FOR ALL ATHLETES

NATALIE RIZZO, MS, RD

NewSeed
PRESS

CONTENTS

INTRODUCTION

I remember the exact moment I understood the phrase "hitting the wall." I signed up to run a half-marathon right before my thirtieth birthday, even though I had never run more than three consecutive miles. I figured it shouldn't be too bad—I was healthy and just like many new (and sometimes experienced) athletes, I thought good overall nutrition would carry me through 13.1 miles. When I did the run, I felt terrible, and I couldn't understand why. I didn't know I needed the extra carbs and sugar that are necessary for long-distance running, and I assumed I drank enough water throughout the day to stay hydrated. I couldn't have been more wrong!

After plenty of research, I finally mastered my fueling routine and came to a realization: Sports nutrition is different from general nutrition. Nutrition is about eating the right nutrients for overall health, but sports nutrition has more nuances, like nutrient timing, meal composition, and hydration. Throw plant-based eating into the mix, and you've got a recipe (pun intended) for confusion.

But I'll let you in on a little secret: Fueling for activity shouldn't be difficult. It can be quite simple once you learn the rules and figure out what works for you. Although I may be biased (I am a registered dietitian after all), I truly believe that nutrition plays as much of a role in performance as training. In fact, choosing the right foods at the right time can enhance your performance, and I'm here to help you figure out what those foods are and when to eat them!

If you think fueling your fitness has to be boring, complicated, or tasteless, think again. Every single recipe in this book is easy to prepare, plant-based, and delicious. Each chapter provides insight about how meal timing plays a role in overall athletic fitness, and the recipes are meant to fuel you through every part of the day.

Chapter 1 discusses everything you need to know about eating a plant-based diet, including nutrients to prioritize and how to get enough protein. Next, dive into what to eat before, during, and after a workout. The question I receive most often is, "What should I eat before my workout?" This chapter answers that question, discusses whether you should add fuel during your workout, and touches on the importance of recovery nutrition.

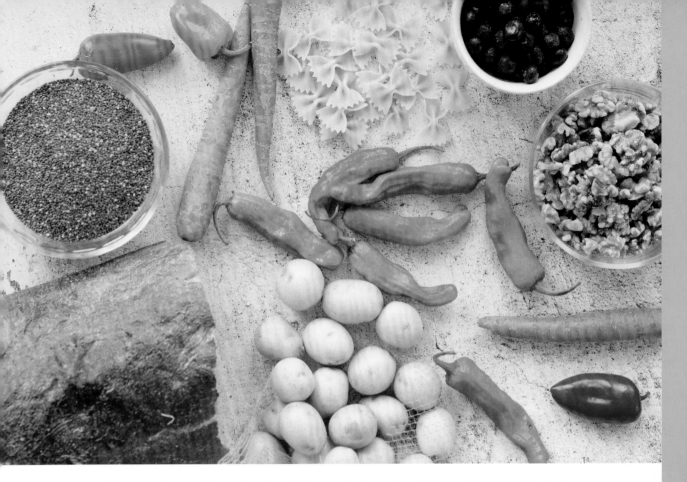

Chapter 2 provides simple, daily meal plans for different types of training days (endurance, intense, strength, and rest), as well as two 7-day meal plans. In addition, there are simple meal-prep tips to make planning your meals easy—because you'd probably rather spend your time training than in the kitchen.

The rest of the book is dedicated to recipes. Each chapter tells you when to incorporate a recipe into your training day. For example, Chapter 3 has preworkout breakfast and snacks, and Chapter 4 is full of lunches that nourish and refuel evening workouts. And the hearty dinners in Chapter 5, easy sides and dips in Chapter 6, and simple desserts in Chapter 7 are sure to become your new everyday staples.

All athletes can benefit from the nutritious recipes in this book, but there is special emphasis on endurance athletes in Chapters 8 and 9. Chapter 8 contains recipes that are meant to be eaten during a workout. You'll find portable recipes that are easy to digest, like sports drinks, energy bites, and homemade jam. Chapter 9 is for anyone who wants to carb load for a race, with recipes that feature pasta, potatoes, rice, and other carb-rich staples. Regardless of the chapter, every single recipe is nutritious, plant-based, and fits perfectly into any training plan!

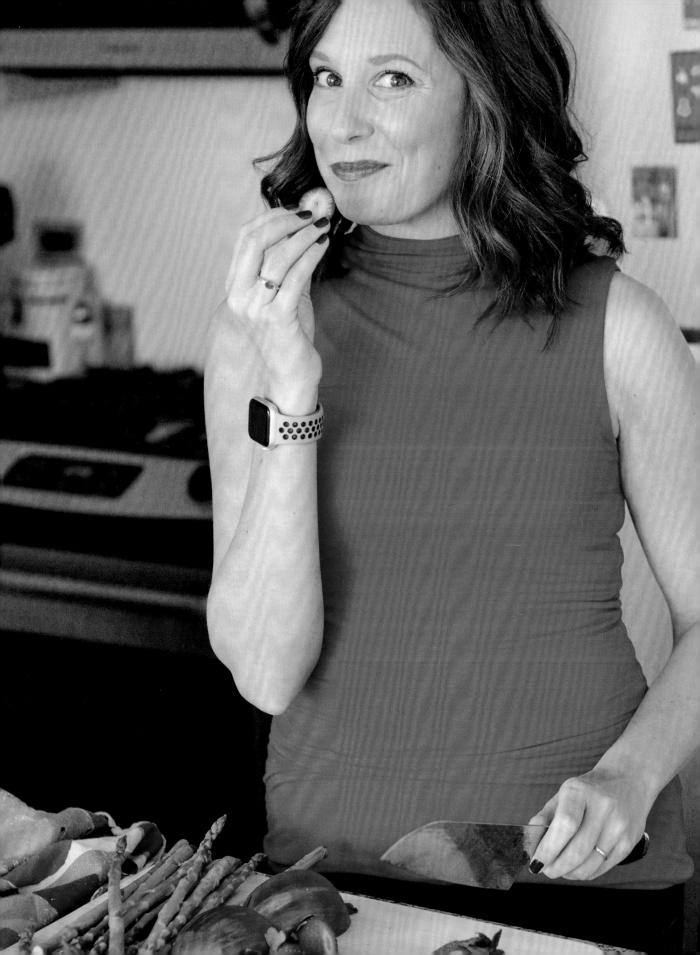

CHAPTER 1

BENEFITS OF A PLANT-BASED DIET

If you bought this book, chances are, you're already on a plant-based diet. Or maybe, you're looking to incorporate more plants into your diet and need a boost! The benefits of plant-based eating for overall health are numerous. Plant-based diets, including vegetarian and vegan diets, have been well studied for their role in disease prevention. Since plant-based diets are rich in whole foods, such as fruits, vegetables, beans, legumes, nuts, soy, seeds, and whole grains, they contain plenty of beneficial nutrients: vitamins, minerals, fiber, and antioxidants. The American Institute for Cancer Research recommends that Americans consume two-thirds of their dietary intake from vegetables, fruits, whole grains, and beans. In the *2015–2020 Dietary Guidelines for Americans*, vegetarian diets are recommended as one of three healthy dietary patterns. Vegetarian diets also improve several heart disease risk factors, including abdominal obesity, blood pressure, blood lipids, and blood glucose. What's more, for those who suffer from risk factors for heart disease, such as high cholesterol, a vegetarian diet may reduce cholesterol levels, decrease markers of inflammation, protect against plaque formation in the arteries, and improve heart health without the use of cholesterol-lowering drugs. Consequently, vegetarians have a reduced risk of developing and dying from heart disease. Researchers attribute these benefits to the abundance of fiber and scarcity of saturated fat (see page 10) in vegetarian and vegan diets. Additionally, compared with meat-eaters, vegetarians and vegans have a lower risk of developing type 2 diabetes and cancer, especially gastro-intestinal cancer.

MACRONUTRIENTS

Let's get into the nitty gritty of what to put in your body, starting with macro-nutrients. There are three macronutrients: (1) carbohydrates, (2) protein, and (3) fat. The body needs macronutrients in large amounts to provide calories and energy for daily functions. Macronutrients in food are not isolated; most foods typically contain all three. The most abundant macronutrient in food determines its classification as a carb, protein, or fat. For example, nuts and seeds contain fat and protein, but they usually fall into the fat category because that nutrient outweighs protein. Beans and lentils are rich in both carbohydrates and protein. Many plant-based eaters eat beans and lentils for protein, while meat-eating athletes that are carb loading may eat them because they are high in carbs. Athletes should understand these macros in order to utilize them to their benefit. Let's look at the roles that carbohy-drates, fat, and protein play on performance.

⫸ Carbohydrates

Carbohydrates are the body's main energy source for exercise and daily functions. The body breaks down all forms of dietary carbs into glucose, a simple sugar that is absorbed into the bloodstream. While some of that simple sugar is used for energy, excess carbs that the body doesn't need right away are stored in the liver and muscles in the form of glycogen, which is the main fuel source for the first 10 to 15 minutes of activity. After glycogen is used, the body turns to any extra carbs floating in the bloodstream to keep energy levels high. Eating preworkout carbs to maintain glycogen and blood glucose can positively impact performance. On the other hand, depletion of these stores is associated with fatigue, impaired skill and concentration, and increased perception of effort.

COMPLEX AND SIMPLE CARBS

When you hear the word "carbs," you may think of not-so-healthy foods, such as desserts, processed snacks, white bread, and sugar. But carbs are also in healthy foods, like whole grains, beans, legumes, dairy, fruits, and vegetables. There are two types of carbohydrates: complex and simple. Complex carbs are made up of long-chain sugar molecules, and simple carbs are small sugar molecules. Because of their long chain, complex carbs take longer to digest and contribute to satiety. In contrast, simple carbs are broken down quickly to provide rapid glucose into the bloodstream.

Both types of carbs are present in many foods. Complex carbs are found in many healthy plant-based foods, such as whole grains, beans, and legumes. Simple carbs, on the other hand, are present in fruit, vegetables, dairy, and sugary foods, such as desserts, syrup, soda, etc. For the non-athlete, choosing mostly complex carbs with plenty of fruits and vegetables and limiting simple carbs from added sugar is a good idea. That said, athletes rely on simple carbs for quick-acting energy for sport. We will discuss this in detail on page 17.

DAILY RECOMMENDED LEVELS

The daily recommendations for carbs are based on a person's activity levels and size. Individuals engaged in a general fitness program should consume about 45 to 55 percent of calories from carbohydrates. That usually equates to about 3 to 5 grams of carbs per kilogram (1.3 to 2.2 grams per pound) of body weight per day. For a 150-pound person, that's roughly 195 to 330 grams of carbs each day.

However, athletes involved in moderate- and high-volume training need greater amounts of carbohydrates in their diet. Those who train for 1 to 3 hours per day of intense exercise five to six times per week should aim for 5 to 8 grams of carbs per kilogram (2.2 to 3.6 grams per pound) of body weight per day. For the same 150-pound athlete, that equals about 330 to 540 grams of carbs each day.

If your training demands are even higher than that—more than 3 hours in one to two daily workouts for five to six days per week—you may need to consume 8 to 10 grams of carbs per kilogram (3.6 to 4.5 grams per pound) of body weight per day. To use the prior example again, that's 540 to 675 daily grams of carbs for a 150-pound athlete. Eating this amount of daily carbs can be grueling and cumbersome. Refer to "Carb-Loading Staples" (see page 151) for meals that will help you reach these daily goals. Don't be scared to include carb-rich beverages, like sports drinks, coconut water, 100 percent fruit juice, and chocolate milk in your carb-loading plan.

⟫⟫ Fat

Fat is a necessary component of a healthy diet, as it provides energy and contributes to cell membranes and the absorption of fat-soluble vitamins. Many people are surprised to learn that at least 20 percent of their daily calories should come from fat. Most athletes should strive to consume 30 percent of their calories from fat, and that number may even reach 50 percent during high-volume training.

SATURATED AND UNSATURATED FAT

There are two types of fat: saturated and unsaturated fat. The difference lies in the chemical structure of the molecule. Saturated fats are often referred to as the "bad" fats, and they are mostly found in animal sources, such as meat, eggs, cheese, butter, and milk. Saturated fat is also prevalent in many desserts, such as cupcakes, pastries, donuts, and candy. Too much saturated fat can cause health problems, such as high cholesterol and heart disease.

Unsaturated fats are known as the "good" fats, and they include omega-3s and omega-6s. The omegas are essential fatty acids—the body needs them for survival, and they can only be obtained by eating food. So-called good fats are usually found in plant sources, such as avocados, nuts, soybeans, seeds, and oils. Many studies have found that a diet rich in good fats can enhance brain function, may lower "bad" (LDL) cholesterol and triglycerides, and can reduce the risk of developing serious diseases, such as heart disease and cancer.

DAILY RECOMMENDED FAT LEVELS

The amount of fat to eat daily has become a source of confusion among athletes because of the recent interest in high-fat and low-carbohydrate diets, such as the ketogenic diet. Some high-performing athletes swear that they can train their bodies to burn fat as fuel, rather than carbohydrates. The present evidence suggests that using fat as fuel not only is inefficient but also may impair performance. Conversely, athletes may choose to excessively restrict their fat intake to lose body weight or improve body composition. Athletes should be discouraged from consuming less than 20 percent of calories from fat, since it limits the variety of nutrients in the diet, such as fat-soluble vitamins and essential fatty acids. As for those "bad" fats, the dietary guidelines recommend eating no more than 10 percent of calories from saturated fat daily.

>>> Protein

Protein plays multiple roles in the body, but for the purposes of this book, we'll focus on its role in muscle building. Although protein is most known for being abundant in animal foods, such as meat, dairy, and eggs, it's also rich in plant-based foods, such as soy, beans, legumes, seeds, and nuts. Some vegetables even contain small amounts of protein. Both protein intake and exercise are necessary for muscle growth and maintenance.

Protein is made up of twenty amino acids, which are organic molecules that combine to form protein. Of those twenty, nine are essential and can only be obtained by eating food. The amino acid distribution profile for plant-based foods is less optimal than for animal foods. Some amino acids are limited in certain plant-based proteins. For example, lysine is present in very small amounts in grains, and methionine and cysteine levels are low in legumes. However, if you're a plant-based eater with a varied diet that consists of many grains, beans, and legumes, you'll still get a healthy dosage of amino acids in your diet.

In the sports world, there is a large emphasis on branched-chain amino acids (BCAAs). These three amino acids—leucine, isoleucine, and valine—have a unique ability to help with muscle building and overall performance. BCAAs may serve as an energy source during a workout, slowing the breakdown of muscle protein. They also help build new muscle after a workout. While many supplements (powders, waters, pills, etc.) contain BCAAs, they are also readily available in certain plant foods. Tofu, quinoa, red lentils, hemp seeds, and peanuts are some of the top whole-food plant sources of BCAAs.

According to the Academy of Nutrition and Dietetics, vegans and vegetarians who eat a variety of plant-based proteins throughout the day should have no problem meeting their protein needs. Research on protein supplements suggests rice and pea protein may stimulate changes in muscle and strength just as well as whey protein.

DAILY RECOMMENDED PROTEIN LEVELS

The recommended daily allowance (RDA) for protein is 0.8 grams per kilogram (0.36 grams per pound) of body weight per day. Although each athlete is different, higher intakes are generally recommended for shorter periods of intense training. A recent meta-analysis found that most athletes benefit from a protein intake of around 1.6 grams per kilogram (0.72 grams per pound) of body weight per day to maintain muscle mass. It's of the utmost importance to ensure you take in enough calories, particularly carbohydrates, to meet energy expenditure. If athletes burn more calories than they consume, their bodies will start to break down lean muscle for use as fuel. Over time, this may lead to muscle wasting, injuries, illness, and training issues.

A DEEPER DIVE INTO PLANT-BASED PROTEIN

Protein is the number one concern among many plant-based athletes. You may wonder if you're getting enough, or you may struggle to understand how much you need daily. Let me assure you that eating enough protein on a plant-based diet is feasible and easy! There are a couple of things you need to understand when it comes to plant-based protein: portion size and protein source.

Generally, you may need to increase portion sizes when cutting meat from your diet. Plant-based foods tend to be lower in calories and protein than animal foods. For example, 3 ounces of tofu have about 10 grams of protein and 90 calories, but 3 ounces of chicken have about 20 grams of protein and 200 calories. You'd need to eat double the amount of tofu to get the same nutrients as chicken. Tofu isn't the only source of protein on a plant-based diet. Whole grains, beans and legumes, soy products, and nuts and seeds are also excellent sources.

⟫⟫ Whole Grains

Whole grains, such as barley, oats, brown rice, farro, spelt, quinoa, and even popcorn, add healthy carbs, protein, and fiber to a plant-based diet. In general, whole grains have more protein than refined grains. The amounts aren't nearly as substantial as soy, beans, legumes, nuts, and seeds, but whole grains can still contribute some protein to a well-balanced meal. Here are some of the top sources of whole grains with plant-based protein, along with their protein content per serving:

- Amaranth (cooked): 6 grams in ⅔ cup
- Oats (dried): 5 grams in ½ cup
- Quinoa (cooked): 8 grams in 1 cup

⋙ Beans and Legumes

Beans and legumes are staples on a plant-based diet and help keep you full long after eating. Stock your pantry with canned beans (black beans, black-eyed peas, white beans, and kidney beans) and legumes (dried lentils, chickpeas, peanuts, and soybeans). Both beans and legumes are rich in fiber, which contributes to heart health and digestion. That said, they also may make you gassy and bloated. It's probably best to work out before eating beans and legumes to avoid an upset stomach. The protein in beans and legumes makes them an excellent postworkout recovery food. Here are some of the top sources of beans and legumes with plant-based protein, along with their protein content per serving:

- Lentils (cooked): 13 grams in ½ cup
- Peanuts: 7 grams in 1 ounce
- Black beans (canned): 7 grams in ½ cup
- Chickpeas (cooked): 6 grams in ½ cup
- Peas (cooked): 5 grams in ⅔ cup

⋙ Soy Products

Some of the best sources of protein on a plant-based diet are soy foods: tofu, tempeh, soy milk, and edamame. These foods are not only inexpensive and easy to cook but also versatile and rich in nutrients. Additionally, soy is a great source of calcium. Plant-based eaters that don't eat dairy need to make sure they get enough of this bone-building mineral from other foods. Some brands of tofu and tempeh are also fortified with vitamin B_{12} and vitamin D to boost their nutrition profile.

Soy also contains isoflavone, a plant compound that possesses estrogen-like qualities. Many people worry about consuming an estrogen-like compound, but research on soy suggests that soy isoflavone intake could lower the risk of breast cancer for both pre- and postmenopausal women and has little to no effect on men. Soy may also help decrease hot flashes for postmenopausal women. Here are some of the top sources of soy foods with plant-based protein, along with their protein content per serving:

- Tempeh: 16 grams in 3 ounces
- Tofu: 9 grams in 3 ounces (one-fifth block)
- Edamame: 9 grams in ½ cup

>>> Nuts and Seeds

Nuts and seeds are a major source of healthy fats for a plant-based diet, and they also contain some protein. All nuts and seeds, such as walnuts, pistachios, almonds, Brazil nuts, macadamia nuts, pecans, chia seeds, sesame seeds, flaxseed, poppy seeds, and hemp seeds, are great additions to your plant-based lifestyle. Many people who are new to plant-based eating worry about hunger levels; to counter that, eat foods with fat and protein to help you feel full. Here are some of the top sources of nuts and seeds with plant-based protein, along with their protein content per serving:

- Hemp seeds: 10 grams in 3 tablespoons
- Pumpkin seeds: 7 grams in 1 ounce
- Almonds: 6 grams in 1 ounce
- Chia seeds: 4 grams in 2 tablespoons
- Walnuts: 4 grams in 1 ounce

MICRONUTRIENTS (TO WATCH)

Micronutrients are vitamins and minerals that come from food. There is a long list of essential vitamins and minerals, and some are less prevalent in plant-based foods. I like to refer to these as "micronutrients to watch." You need to put in a bit more effort to make sure you don't end up with a deficiency, but it's not difficult to do once you get into a habit of it! The three plant-based micronutrients to watch are (1) iron, (2) calcium, and (3) vitamin B_{12}.

>>> Iron

Iron is a mineral that is used in the human body to make oxygen-carrying proteins. It also plays a role in physical growth, neurological development, cellular functioning, and the synthesis of some hormones. There are two forms of iron: heme and non-heme. Heme iron comes from the blood of animals and is only found in animal foods: poultry, fish, beef, and pork. This form of iron is most easily absorbed by the body. On the other hand, non-heme iron is found in plant sources, such as grains, fortified cereals, beans, nuts, seeds, and vegetables. Non-heme iron is not as well absorbed by the body, and you need more of it to meet your iron needs. Some of the best sources of non-heme iron are chickpeas, spinach, oats, tofu, lentils, potatoes, cashews, edamame, sesame seeds, flaxseed, beets, and white mushrooms.

The recommended daily allowance (RDA) for iron is different for men and women. Men ages 19–50 need 8 milligrams of iron per day, while women of the same age need 18 milligrams. Both men and women over 51 need 8 milligrams of iron per day. The National Institutes of Health (NIH) recommends that vegetarians eat 1.8 times more iron than meat-eaters, which is about 14 milligrams for men and 32 milligrams for women.

Evidence on vegetarian athletes and long-distance runners shows that they are at greater risk for developing an iron deficiency due to losses in urine, sweat, and feces. Athletes that are diagnosed with iron deficiency anemia should speak to their doctor before taking a supplement. Iron supplementation can improve athletic performance, but unmonitored supplementation is not recommended; too much iron in the blood can be toxic.

>>> Calcium

Most known for its role in maintaining strong bones, calcium is also stored in the teeth and plays a role in structure and hardness. Calcium is also used for blood clotting, sending and receiving nerve signals, squeezing and relaxing muscles, releasing hormones and other chemicals, and maintaining a normal heartbeat.

Men and women ages 19–50 need 1,000 milligrams of calcium per day, while everyone over 50 needs 1,200 milligrams per day. This important mineral is most prevalent in dairy foods, with 300 milligrams (30 percent of daily value) in a glass of milk and 240 milligrams (24 percent of daily value) in 7 ounces of Greek yogurt. Most vegetarians meet or exceed their calcium needs each day, but intakes can vary widely for vegans. Luckily, you can get plenty of calcium from nondairy sources, such as white beans, edamame, tofu, chia seeds, collard greens, kale, butternut squash, almonds, figs, tahini, and fortified orange juice.

Without proper calcium intake, athletes may be at risk for low bone-mineral density and stress fractures, as well as menstrual dysfunction in female athletes. If you have a calcium deficiency, your doctor may recommend taking up to 1,500 milligrams in a supplement per day to optimize bone health.

>>> Vitamin B$_{12}$

Vitamin B$_{12}$ is most known for its role in energy production. This B vitamin contributes to the proper formation of red blood cells, nerves, and DNA. While vitamin B$_{12}$ is abundant in animal products, plants, on the other hand, can't produce vitamin B$_{12}$. Consequently, you won't find much vitamin B$_{12}$ in plant-based foods. There are some rare instances of fermented foods, like tempeh, nori, spirulina, algae, and unfortified nutritional yeast, that do have natural vitamin B$_{12}$ from the process of fermentation, but it's best not to rely on getting enough vitamin B$_{12}$ from these fermented foods. Instead, seek out plant foods that are fortified with vitamin B$_{12}$. Fortified plant foods include nutritional yeast, plant milks, meat substitutes, and breakfast cereals. For vegetarians, milk and eggs also provide natural vitamin B$_{12}$, but only about two-thirds the amount you need each day.

Men and women over nineteen years old need 2.4 micrograms (mcg) of vitamin B$_{12}$ per day. The Academy of Nutrition and Dietetics recommends that vegetarians and vegans take precautionary measures to get enough vitamin B$_{12}$. A vitamin B$_{12}$ deficiency can cause unusual fatigue, tingling in fingers and toes, poor cognition, and digestive issues, none of which are ideal for athletes. Inadequate vitamin B$_{12}$ intake has been linked to low bone mineral density, increased fracture risk, and osteoporosis. All vegetarians and vegans should be screened for a vitamin B$_{12}$ deficiency through a simple blood test. Most vegans should supplement with 250 micrograms of vitamin B$_{12}$ every day, while vegetarians should consider taking a 250-microgram B$_{12}$ supplement a few times per week.

WHAT TO EAT AND DRINK BEFORE, DURING, AND AFTER A WORKOUT

Now that you've got the macronutrients down, it's time to combine them into meals to fuel your workouts. The chapters in this book are titled in a way that will help you know when to eat what food, but it's still important to understand ideal nutrient timings. Having a good understanding of what to eat before, during, and after a workout can help you build a quick and simple meal when you don't have time to cook or follow a recipe. And trust me, a small tweak to your fueling routine can make a big difference. So, if macronutrients are the "who" of fueling, meal timing is the "when, what, and why."

⟫⟫ Preworkout Nutrition

Since carbs are the primary energy source for exercise, they are a crucial component of the preworkout meal and snack. It takes about 4 hours for carbohydrates to be digested and assimilated into muscle and liver tissues as glycogen. As such, the preworkout meal should occur 4 to 6 hours before exercising. If an athlete trains in the afternoon, a well-balanced breakfast with carbs, protein, and healthy fats can top off muscle and liver glycogen levels.

For athletes who exercise in the morning, a preworkout meal may not be feasible. Instead, a light carbohydrate and protein snack 30 to 60 minutes before exercise (30 to 50 grams of carbohydrate and 5 to 10 grams of protein) can provide quick-acting energy to the muscles. The protein also decreases exercise-induced muscle breakdown and minimizes muscle damage. Choose foods that are lower in fiber to reduce the risk of gastrointestinal issues during the event. Simple carbs are digested more quickly, making them the perfect option for preworkout snacking. Some practical solutions for quick fueling include:

- Cereal
- Dried fruit, like dates
- Fresh fruit, like a banana or apple
- Granola
- Sports drink, gel, or gummies
- Toast with nut butter

⟫⟫ During Workout Nutrition

Believe it or not, there are instances when you need to take in fuel during a workout. Just like preworkout nutrition, the timing and amount of fuel you ingest during a workout depends on a few factors. First, glycogen and dietary carbs are the main fuel source for exercise, and they both work to limit fatigue for about 60 minutes. However, during a sustained high-intensity workout of 45 to 75 minutes, the body may need extra fuel to keep energy levels high. In this situation, a few small sips of a sports drink provide easily digested carbs for quick energy.

During endurance exercise lasting 60 minutes to 2.5 hours, it's necessary to fuel with 30 to 60 grams of carbohydrates per hour after the first 60 minutes. Sports products, like sports drinks, gummies, and gels are specifically designed to provide rapidly digested carbs the body needs in these times. In addition, many of them provide multiple sources of carbohydrates, like glucose and fructose, which have been shown to have higher rates of digestion during endurance activity.

If you prefer natural fuel during a workout, opt for simple carbs that digest quickly and add a dash of salt to replace sodium losses from sweat. Make sure you also drink water throughout the entire workout to stay hydrated. See the list of natural foods below that are rich in sugar and low in fiber. Check the nutrition facts label and measure out portions that have about 30 grams of carbohydrates, then add a dash of salt to each option.

- Applesauce
- Dates or raisins
- Fresh fruit, like a banana
- Gummy bears or jelly beans
- Homemade sports drinks
- Maple syrup or honey packet

- Mashed sweet potatoes
- Pretzels
- Unsweetened cereal, like Corn Flakes or Cheerios
- White bread with jam
- White crackers, like saltines

≫ Postworkout Recovery

During a workout, two things occur within the body that warrant recovery nutrition: (1) the muscles experience tiny tears, and (2) carbohydrate stores are depleted. Postworkout protein is necessary to repair the worn-down muscle tissue, while carbohydrates restock glycogen in the muscle and liver. Both protein and carbohydrates not only make you feel stronger after a workout but also fight off fatigue and prepare the body for another workout.

Following intense exercise, it's recommended that you consume 0.25 to 0.3 grams of protein per kilogram of body weight, or 15 to 25 grams of protein. This range fits most athletes with average body sizes, but the recommendations may need to be adjusted for those at extreme ends of the weight spectrum. Doses exceeding 40 grams of postworkout protein have not yet been shown to further stimulate muscle protein synthesis. In addition, research suggests that a 3:1 carb to protein ratio is ideal for recovery. That means consuming 1 gram of protein for every 3 grams of carbs. For example, a postworkout snack may have 8 grams of protein and 24 grams of carbohydrates.

After immediate postworkout recovery nutrition, eat a well-balanced meal with carbs, protein, and fat within 2 hours after exercise. Studies in resistance-trained athletes show an increased rate of muscle protein synthesis for at least 24 hours after exercise. In other words, recovery nutrition lasts for an entire day, not just a few hours. Not to mention that eating well-balanced meals throughout the day satiates hunger and prevents overeating.

>>> Hydration

Being hydrated during athletic activity plays a large role in overall performance. Humans lose water through respiration, the gastrointestinal system, kidneys, and sweat. Losing too much water may cause a loss in blood volume, which can lead to cardiovascular strain, increased glycogen use, altered metabolic and central nervous system function, and a greater rise in body temperature. In addition to water, sweat contains the electrolytes sodium, potassium, calcium, and magnesium. Although every individual is different, it's generally accepted that fluid deficits of more than 2 percent of body weight can compromise cognitive function and performance, particularly in hot weather. Most athletes finish exercising with a fluid deficit and need to rehydrate immediately following a workout. Rehydration strategies are simple: Drink water and take in some sodium.

To prevent dehydration, athletes should consume 5 to 10 milliliters (mL) of fluid per kilogram (2 to 4 milliliters per pound) of body weight in the 2 to 4 hours before exercise. You'll be able to tell that you're properly hydrated if your urine is pale yellow, as opposed to dark yellow, which signifies dehydration. In addition, sodium should be ingested during exercise by athletes who have high sweat rates, salty sweat, or exercise for 90 minutes or more. Although skeletal muscle cramps are typically caused by muscle fatigue, they may come from dehydration and electrolyte imbalances. If you experience cramps regularly, look at your hydration routine to see if it's the culprit.

Drinking more fluid than you sweat can cause hyponatremia, also known as water intoxication. This is compounded by excessive fluid intake in the hours or days leading up to the event. If you are drinking excessively, your urine is clear—rather than pale yellow—and you start to experience nausea, dizziness, loss of energy, or muscle weakness, seek medical help immediately.

MOVING FORWARD

By following the principles you've learned in this chapter and looking at the sample meal plans in the next, you'll be on your way to building a meal plan that works for your sport. Pair that with the yummy recipes in the remaining chapters and fueling will start to feel like fun rather than a chore.

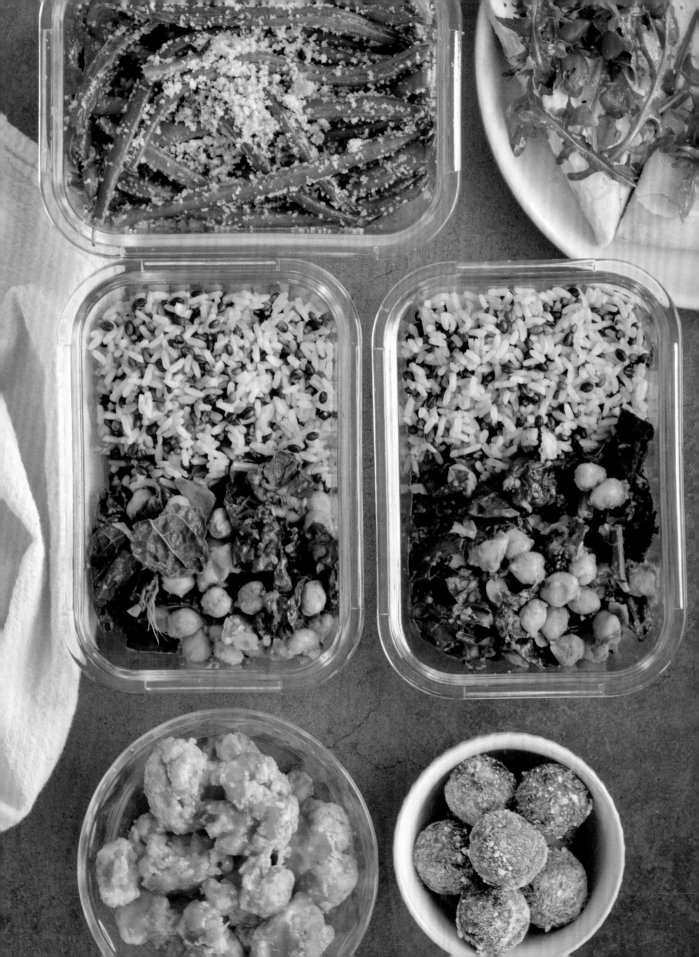

CHAPTER 2

MEAL PLANS

Although the following chapters are full of healthy plant-based recipes, linking them together into a cohesive menu that works for your training demands can be tricky. This chapter solves that problem! Here you'll find examples of what to eat on four different types of training days (endurance, intense, strength, and rest), as well as a two 7-day meal plans. If you eat healthy well-balanced meals on any type of training day, you'll be setting yourself up for success. But to take it the next level, there are nuances to consider. For instance, eat more calories and carbs on intense days and up the protein intake on strength-training days. Since meal plans can seem a bit overwhelming, I've included my best meal prep tips at the end of this chapter to get you started.

ENDURANCE-TRAINING DAY

This sample day is formulated for the athlete who spends about 60 minutes or less engaging in endurance activity. The meals are well balanced to include carbs, protein, and fat, as well as a variety of vitamins, minerals, and antioxidants. Most of the meals are moderate in calories; you may need more or fewer calories than these meals provide based on your size and activity level. Start your day with a simple muesli that contains fiber-rich oats, nuts, and seeds, and pair it with a protein, like yogurt or soy milk. Then whip up a wrap for lunch, which has carbs from the wrap, protein from the chickpeas, and healthy fat from the avocado. This combo will keep you full for hours, but don't forget to eat a simple snack to top off your fuel stores. Dip your favorite veggies in the homemade ranch dip. End the day with one of my favorite dinner options: either cauliflower tacos or a mushroom burger. And since the desserts in this book are quick, easy, and on the healthier side, feel free to indulge in a slice of cake. No matter what time of the day you work out, you'll have plenty of gas in the tank from the combination of nutrients in each meal.

Breakfast	Pumpkin Pie Muesli (page 38)
Lunch	Chickpea Avocado Smash Wrap (page 57)
Snack	Veggies + Yogurt Ranch Dip (page 100)
Dinner Option 1	Cauliflower Tacos with Chipotle Crema (page 86)
Dinner Option 2	Wild Rice and Mushroom Umami Burgers with Roasted Red Pepper Aioli (page 90) + Rosemary Roasted Delicata Squash (page 113)
Dessert (optional)	Lemon Cake (page 134)

INTENSE-TRAINING DAY

Intense-training days consist of more than 60 minutes of endurance activity, such as a long run, cycle, or swim. For the student or professional athlete, this may include race day or game day. There are three main goals for fueling an intense-training day. First, make sure you take in plenty of carbs before the activity to top off glycogen and make your energy last. Second, eat easy-to-digest carbs during the activity to keep your energy levels high when glycogen runs out. Third, recover properly after training with carbs to replace glycogen, protein to aid in muscle repair, and healthy fats to satisfy hunger. To account for these changes, this sample day has meals that are slightly higher in carbs and includes workout fuel to eat during training. Start your day with a cold brew smoothie for an extra caffeine jolt and a slice of quick bread for fast-acting carbs. Pack some date balls to eat during the workout. The dates and pretzels provide the carbs you need to power you through the intense activity and give you a sodium boost to replace electrolytes lost in sweat. Recover with a farro bowl and breakfast cookies. End the day with a hearty dinner, like the ravioli bowl or stuffed butternut squash. Top off your day with a serving of fruit crisp.

Breakfast	Cold Brew Oat Milk Smoothie (page 34) + Key Lime Quick Bread (page 48)
During Workout Fuel	Sweet and Salty Pretzel Date Bites (page 145)
Lunch	Fall Sweet Potato, Apple, Kale, and Farro Bowl (page 67)
Snack	Almond Butter Chocolate Chip Breakfast Cookies (page 41)
Dinner Option 1	Mediterranean Ravioli Bowl (page 163)
Dinner Option 2	Stuffed Butternut Squash with Sorghum (page 171) + Sweet Chile Brussels Sprouts (page 109)
Dessert (optional)	Plum Crisp (page 133)

STRENGTH-TRAINING DAY

Strength training contributes to muscle protein synthesis and increased power output, as well as injury prevention. Most endurance athletes strength train at least a few times each week, and their carb and calorie needs are slightly lower on these days. That doesn't mean you should go low carb or restrict calories, but you should focus on a bit more protein to aid in muscle recovery after a heavy strength session. Muscles grow stronger in the recovery phase, so nourishing them with protein increases overall endurance. This strength-training meal plan includes some of the higher protein meals in this book. Breakfast starts with a smoothie, made with silken tofu, as well as a little bit of carbs in the pie bites. The gyro is one of the most well-rounded and delicious lunches, with ample protein from the tempeh (a fermented soybean). Have a handful or two of muesli for a snack, as it's got plenty of protein from the nuts and seeds. Finish the day with tofu or "meatballs," both of which pack a protein punch. If you'd like a sweet end cap, try the no-added-sugar chia seed pudding.

Breakfast	Black Forest Smoothie (page 35) + Apple Pie Bites (page 37)
Lunch	Tempeh Gyro with Tofu Tzatziki Sauce (page 60)
Snack	Pumpkin Pie Muesli (page 38)
Dinner Option 1	Sweet and Sticky Tofu (page 85) + Garlicky Green Beans (page 107)
Dinner Option 2	Spaghetti Squash with Lentil "Meatballs" (page 94)
Dessert (optional)	Tropical Chia Seed Pudding (page 123)

REST DAY

Contrary to popular belief, you should not drastically cut calories on a rest day. The body recovers while resting, which means that you need to take in well-balanced meals to grow stronger and prepare for the next day's workout. That's why the rest day plan looks very similar to the normal training day or strength-training day. Take in a balance of carbs to replenish glycogen, protein to help tired muscles recover, and healthy fats to control hunger. You might want to skip dessert on a rest day, but otherwise eat plenty of food. Whip up a smoothie for breakfast with a handful of healthy fats, like candied walnuts. A quesadilla is the perfect well-balanced lunch, and it takes just minutes to make. Make a batch of the chia jam to snack on with crackers for a quick healthy snack. Finish the day with a big bowl of soup or chili.

Breakfast	Blueberry and Cinnamon Apple Smoothie (page 44) + Candied Maple Ginger Walnuts (page 45)
Lunch	Black Bean Quesadillas (page 63)
Snack	Homemade Strawberry Chia Jam (page 141) + crackers
Dinner Option 1	Greens and Beans Soup (page 78)
Dinner Option 2	Pumpkin Chili (page 81)

PUTTING IT ALL TOGETHER

I've put together two 7-day meal plans to show what an average training week might look like. The first is a meal plan for moderate training needs. This is for the athlete who isn't training for a long-distance event and doesn't have an intense day in their training schedule. Think of this as maintenance mode or as a way of eating healthy meals in your off-season. The second meal plan is for intense training and includes workout fuel to take in during exercise and a bit more dessert. Naturally, this meal plan is higher in calories to make up for the ones you're expending. Take note of that!

⟫⟫ Moderate-Training Plan

MEAL	MONDAY (Endurance Training)	TUESDAY (Strength Training)	WEDNESDAY (Endurance Training)
Breakfast	Pumpkin Pie Muesli (page 38)	Black Forest Smoothie (page 35) + Apple Pie Bites (page 37)	*Leftover* Pumpkin Pie Muesli
Lunch	Chickpea Avocado Smash Wrap (page 57)	Tempeh Gyro with Tofu Tzatziki Sauce (page 60)	*Leftover* Chickpea Avocado Smash Wrap
Snack	Veggies + Yogurt Ranch Dip (page 100)	*Leftover* Pumpkin Pie Muesli	*Leftover* veggies + Yogurt Ranch Dip
Dinner	Cauliflower Tacos with Chipotle Crema (page 86)	Sweet and Sticky Tofu (page 85) + Garlicky Green Beans (page 107)	*Leftover* Cauliflower Tacos with Chipotle Crema
Dessert	Lemon Cake (page 134)	Tropical Chia Seed Pudding (page 123)	*Leftover* Lemon Cake

THURSDAY (Rest Day)	FRIDAY (Endurance Training)	SATURDAY (Strength Training)	SUNDAY (Rest Day)
Blueberry and Cinnamon Apple Smoothie (page 44) + Candied Maple Ginger Walnuts (page 45)	*Leftover* Pumpkin Pie Muesli	*Leftover* Black Forest Smoothie + *Leftover* Apple Pie Bites	*Leftover* Blueberry and Cinnamon Apple Smoothie + *Leftover* Candied Maple Ginger Walnuts
Black Bean Quesadillas (page 63)	*Leftover* Chickpea Avocado Smash Wrap	*Leftover* Tempeh Gyro with Tofu Tzatziki Sauce	*Leftover* Black Bean Quesadillas
Homemade Strawberry Chia Jam (page 141) + crackers	*Leftover* veggies + Yogurt Ranch Dip	*Leftover* Homemade Strawberry Chia Jam + crackers	*Leftover* Homemade Strawberry Chia Jam + crackers
Greens and Beans Soup (page 78)	*Leftover* Cauliflower Tacos with Chipotle Crema	*Leftover* Sweet and Sticky Tofu + *Leftover* Garlicky Green Beans	*Leftover* Greens and Beans Soup
	Leftover Lemon Cake	*Leftover* Tropical Chia Seed Pudding	

⟫ Intense-Training Meal Plan

MEAL	MONDAY (Endurance Training)	TUESDAY (Strength Training)	WEDNESDAY (Intense Training)
Breakfast	Whole Wheat Banana Nut Muffins (page 47)	Black Forest Smoothie (page 35) + Avocado Yogurt Ciabatta Bread (page 51)	Cold Brew Oat Milk Smoothie (page 34) + Key Lime Quick Bread (page 48)
During Workout Fuel			Sweet and Salty Pretzel Date Bites (page 145)
Lunch	Chickpea Avocado Smash Wrap (page 57)	Crumbled Tofu Rancheros (page 75)	Fall Sweet Potato, Apple, Kale and Farro Bowl (page 67)
Snack	Corn and Red Pepper Salsa (page 103) + chips	Pumpkin Pie Muesli (page 38)	Almond Butter Chocolate Chip Breakfast Cookies (page 41)
Dinner	Wild Rice and Mushroom Umami Burgers with Roasted Red Pepper Aioli (page 90) + Rosemary Roasted Delicata Squash (page 113)	Spaghetti Squash with Lentil "Meatballs" (page 94)	Mediterranean Ravioli Bowl (page 163)
Dessert	Baked Pears with Apple Cider Glaze (page 124)	Cinnamon and Sugar Roasted Chickpeas (page 119)	Salted Tahini Chocolate Chip Cookies (page 130)

THURSDAY (Endurance Training)	FRIDAY (Strength Training)	SATURDAY (Intense Training)	SUNDAY (Rest Day)
Leftover Whole Wheat Banana Nut Muffins	Black Forest Smoothie (page 35) + *Leftover* Avocado Yogurt Ciabatta Bread	Cold Brew Oat Milk Smoothie (page 34) + *Leftover* Key Lime Quick Bread	Black Forest Smoothie (page 35) + *Leftover* Avocado Yogurt Ciabatta Bread
		Leftover Sweet and Salty Pretzel Date Bites	
Leftover Chickpea Avocado Smash Wrap	*Leftover* Crumbled Tofu Rancheros	*Leftover* Fall Sweet Potato, Apple, Kale, and Farro Bowl	*Leftover* Crumbled Tofu Rancheros
Leftover Corn and Red Pepper Salsa + chips	*Leftover* Pumpkin Pie Muesli	*Leftover* Almond Butter Chocolate Chip Breakfast Cookies	Homemade Strawberry Chia Jam (page 141) + crackers
Leftover Wild Rice and Mushroom Umami Burgers with Roasted Red Pepper Aioli + *Leftover* Rosemary Roasted Delicata Squash	*Leftover* Spaghetti Squash with Lentil "Meatballs"	*Leftover* Mediterranean Ravioli Bowl	*Leftover* Spaghetti Squash with Lentil "Meatballs"
Leftover Baked Pears with Apple Cider Glaze	*Leftover* Cinnamon and Sugar Roasted Chickpeas	*Leftover* Salted Tahini Chocolate Chip Cookies	

MEAL PREP TIPS

With training demands, work, school, and life, it's not always easy to find time in the kitchen each day. And while the recipes in this book were created with that in mind, utilizing these simple meal prep tips will help you cook multiple meals at once. Meal prepping saves you time and is a great way to ensure that you always have meals and snacks on hand to fuel for and recover from your training. Plus, having healthy prepped meals cuts down on takeout bills. Here are some simple suggestions to make meal prepping a little bit easier.

⫸ Make a Plan

The first step to meal prepping is to start with a plan. Set aside 10 minutes to create a plan for the week. What days will you eat at home? What days will you eat out? What meals do you want to prep? What meals can you make on the fly? After you've thought through your meal prep strategy, choose a few meals to prep. Spoiler alert: You don't have to prep every single meal for the week at once. If you're new to meal prepping, start with two or three meals. You can always add more meals as you feel more comfortable. To cut down on grocery bills and food waste, choose recipes with similar ingredients. For example, if you're buying tofu for Sweet and Sticky Tofu (page 85), add Crumbled Tofu Rancheros (page 75) to your meal plan.

⫸ Buy No-Prep Ingredients

If the thought of chopping veggies or cooking grains is too much for you, buy low-prep or no-prep ingredients. One of the best things about plant-based foods is the ease of preparation. Canned beans are inexpensive and can be rinsed and served immediately. Tofu and tempeh can be eaten right out of the container, although they taste much better when marinated and used in a recipe. Frozen fruits and vegetables can be used in soups and smoothie recipes. Since they're frozen at the peak of freshness, all their nutrients are sealed in. If you don't mind spending a few extra dollars, you can also buy prechopped veggies to save time. The same goes for frozen grains, like quinoa or brown rice. Rather than cook dried grains, you can opt for a bag of the frozen variety and microwave it.

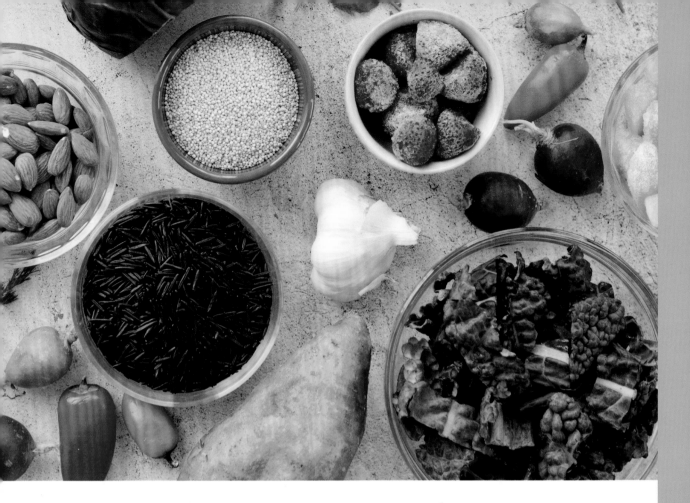

⫸ Multitask

When it's time to start cooking, multitasking is key. Always start with the steps that require more time, such as roasting veggies or cooking grains. If several recipes have the same cooking methods, such as chopping and then roasting in the oven, do both of those steps at the same time. The trick is to have several things cooking at once and compile everything in the end.

⫸ Use Containers

Once everything is prepared, store it in single-serving containers. Any airtight container will do, but I recommend glass single-serving containers for meals, mason jars for drinks and sauces, and reusable plastic bags for odds and ends, such as dressings or toppings. Feel free to also use plastic, if it's microwave-able. All of these steps may seem like a lot of work, but trust me that you'll be so happy you put in the hours when you can pull a fully formed meal from the fridge after a long training session.

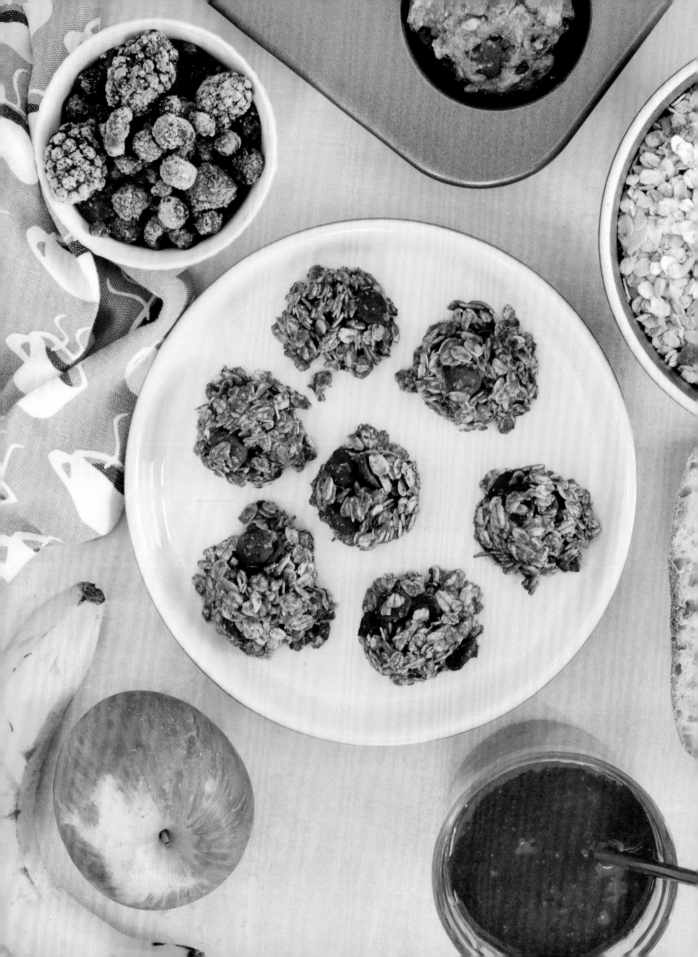

CHAPTER 3

PREWORKOUT BREAKFAST AND SNACKS

These simple snacks and meals are easy to prep ahead or throw together before a morning workout. The recipes are designed to have plenty of easily digestible carbs, making them the perfect preworkout fuel. If you break a sweat before the sun rises and only want a few bites of food, opt for something simple, such as the Apple Pie Bites (page 37) or a Cold Brew Oat Milk Smoothie (page 34). Or if you prefer a slightly bigger preworkout meal, the Raspberry Oat Bars (page 42) or Pumpkin Pie Muesli (page 38) will fill you up without weighing you down.

COLD BREW OAT MILK SMOOTHIE

MAKES 2 SERVINGS • **PREP TIME: 5 MINUTES**

Caffeine before a workout has been shown to increase athletic performance. This smoothie serves two purposes—provide a preworkout jolt and put a little fuel in your stomach. For those who can't tolerate a big meal before a workout, a smoothie is a great option for taking in some easy-to-digest calories. Cold brew is made from soaking ground coffee in water overnight. Luckily, a premade version of this coffee staple is bottled and sold at most supermarkets. Combine the cold brew with creamy oat milk, sweet dates, and ice for a quick, easy smoothie.

8 ounces cold brew

16 ounces unsweetened oat milk

4 Medjool dates, pitted

2 ice cubes

In a blender, combine the cold brew, oat milk, dates, and ice cubes. Blend until smooth.

PER SERVING: Calories: 220, Fat: 4.5g, Sat Fat: 0g, Sodium: 95mg, Carbohydrates: 41g, Dietary Fiber: 4g, Added Sugar: 12g, Protein: 4g, Vitamin D: 3mcg, Calcium: 355mg, Iron: 1mg, Potassium: 697mg

Fun Facts

Research suggests drinking a cup of black coffee before exercise can boost performance. Caffeine takes about 10 minutes to enter the blood stream and typically peaks at about 45 to 75 minutes after ingestion.

BLACK FOREST SMOOTHIE

MAKES 2 SERVINGS • **PREP TIME: 5 MINUTES**

This chocolate-cherry smoothie has a secret ingredient that makes it creamy without dairy—silken tofu. This soft tofu variety has a neutral flavor that blends really well into smoothies, sauces, and dips. It's combined with frozen cherries, cocoa powder, almond milk, and a dash of maple syrup for a rich, velvety smoothie that has plenty of plant-based carbs and protein to keep you full during a workout.

2 cups frozen cherries

⅔ cup silken tofu

1 cup unsweetened almond milk or plant milk of choice

2 tablespoons unsweetened cocoa powder

2 teaspoons maple syrup (optional)

In a blender, combine the cherries, tofu, almond milk, cocoa powder, and maple syrup, if using. Blend until smooth.

PER SERVING: Calories: 130, Fat: 4.5g, Sat Fat: 0.5g, Sodium: 105mg, Carbohydrates: 22g, Dietary Fiber: 4g, Added Sugar: 0g, Protein: 7g, Vitamin D: 1mcg, Calcium: 330mg, Iron: 3mg, Potassium: 508mg

Fun Facts

Unlike juicing, blending fruits and vegetables doesn't destroy the fiber. A smoothie can add fiber, protein, vitamins, minerals, and antioxidants to the diet.

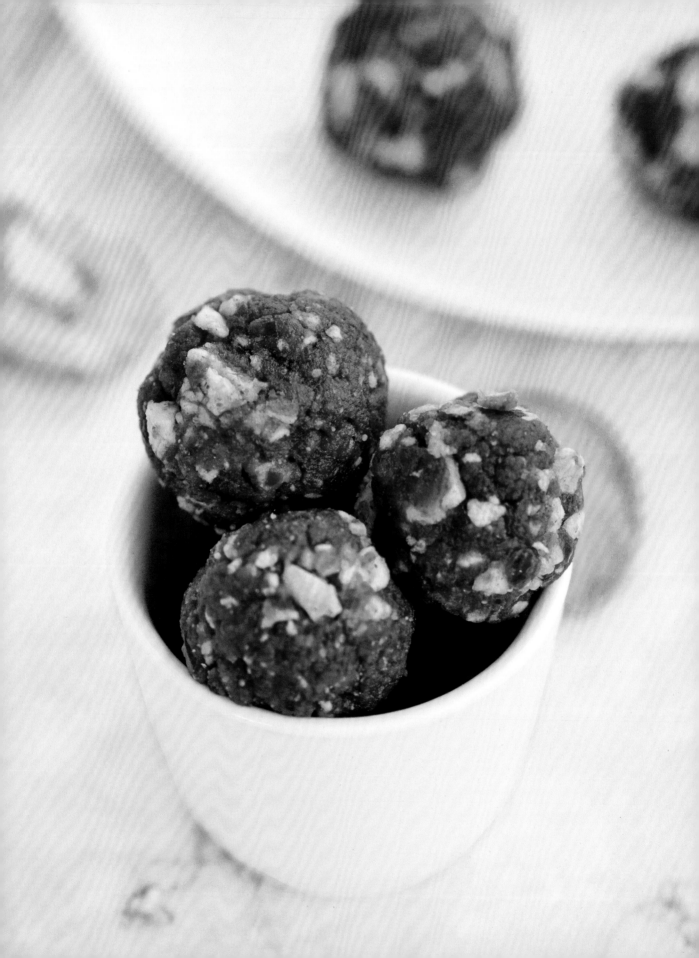

APPLE PIE BITES

MAKES 12 BITES • **PREP TIME: 1 HOUR 5 MINUTES**

These energy bites embody the tastes of fall with dried apple rings and cinnamon. The combination of apple rings and dates provides quick-acting carbs that make these bites great for a digestible preworkout snack. There's no baking required for the taste of apple pie. Just pop all the ingredients in a food processor, blend, refrigerate, and enjoy!

½ cup dried apple rings

½ cup pitted whole dates

½ cup nut butter of choice

I teaspoon ground cinnamon

I tablespoon water

Line a large plate with parchment paper. In a food processor, combine the apple rings, dates, nut butter, cinnamon, and water. Process until you have a paste.

Using your hands, roll the paste into golf ball–size balls.

Place the bites on the prepared plate, leaving some space in between each bite. Refrigerate for at least 1 hour. Serve cold. Store leftover bites in a sealed container in the fridge for up to 7 days.

PER SERVING (2 BITES): Calories: 180, Fat: 11g, Sat Fat: 2g, Sodium: 95mg, Carbohydrates: 20g, Dietary Fiber: 3g, Added Sugar: 1g, Protein: 5g, Vitamin D: 0mcg, Calcium: 21mg, Iron: 1mg, Potassium: 250mg

Fun Facts

Switch up this recipe with any type of dried fruit and nut butter you want! Use cashew butter and dried mango for a tropical twist. Or try dried figs and almond butter for something different.

PUMPKIN PIE MUESLI

MAKES 4 SERVINGS • PREP TIME: 5 MINUTES / COOK TIME: 10 MINUTES

My family loves a good muesli, and I find that making it at home is healthier and cheaper than the store-bought version. A simple mixture of toasted oats, nuts, seeds, dried fruit, and spices, homemade muesli is the perfect preworkout fuel to eat by the handful. Or combine it with yogurt or milk to have after a workout for a quick recovery snack. This version highlights the spices of pumpkin pie with pumpkin seeds for an autumn-inspired dish that cooks in just 10 minutes flat.

1 cup rolled oats

½ cup unsalted sliced raw almonds

⅓ cup unsalted pumpkin seeds

1 teaspoon ground cinnamon

¼ teaspoon ground nutmeg

¼ teaspoon ground allspice

¼ teaspoon salt

⅓ cup dried cranberries

Preheat the oven to 325°F. Line a large baking sheet with parchment paper.

In a large bowl, combine the oats, almonds, pumpkin seeds, cinnamon, nutmeg, allspice, and salt. Stir to combine.

Spread the mixture out evenly on the prepared baking sheet and bake for 10 minutes or until the oats become golden.

Remove the mixture from the oven and add the dried cranberries. Serve warm. Store leftover muesli in a sealed container at room temperature for up to 7 days.

PER SERVING: Calories: 280, Fat: 13g, Sat Fat: 2g, Sodium: 150mg, Carbohydrates: 29g, Dietary Fiber: 6g, Added Sugar: 7g, Protein: 10g, Vitamin D: 0mcg, Calcium: 59mg, Iron: 3mg, Potassium: 164mg

Fun Facts

Seeds are a great way to add protein to a plant-based meal. Add 2 tablespoons of hemp seeds to any grain bowl for an extra 6 grams of protein.

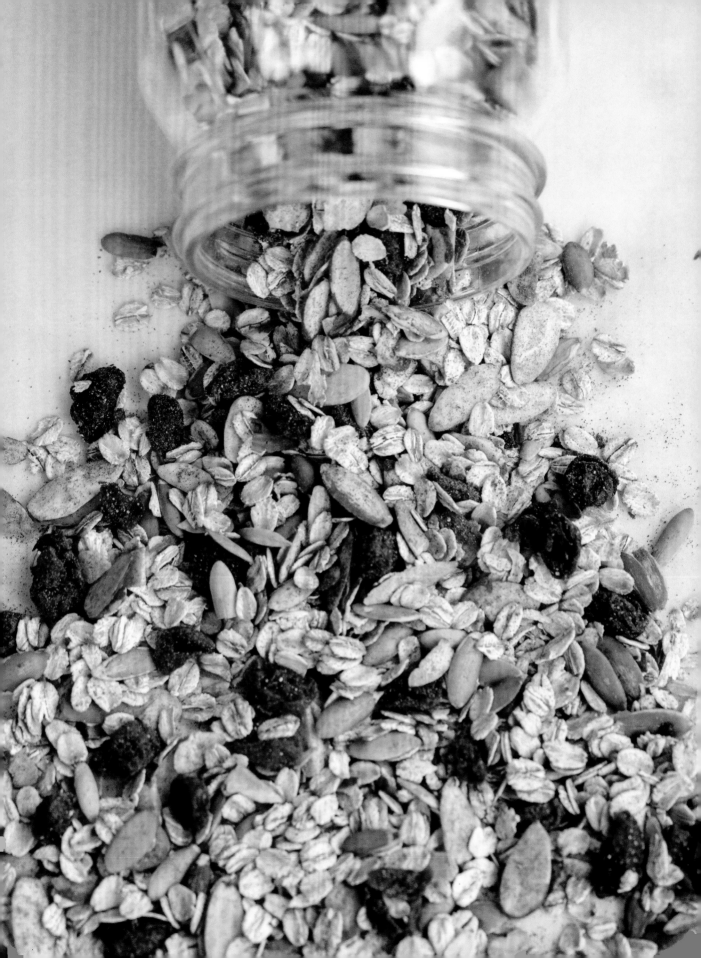

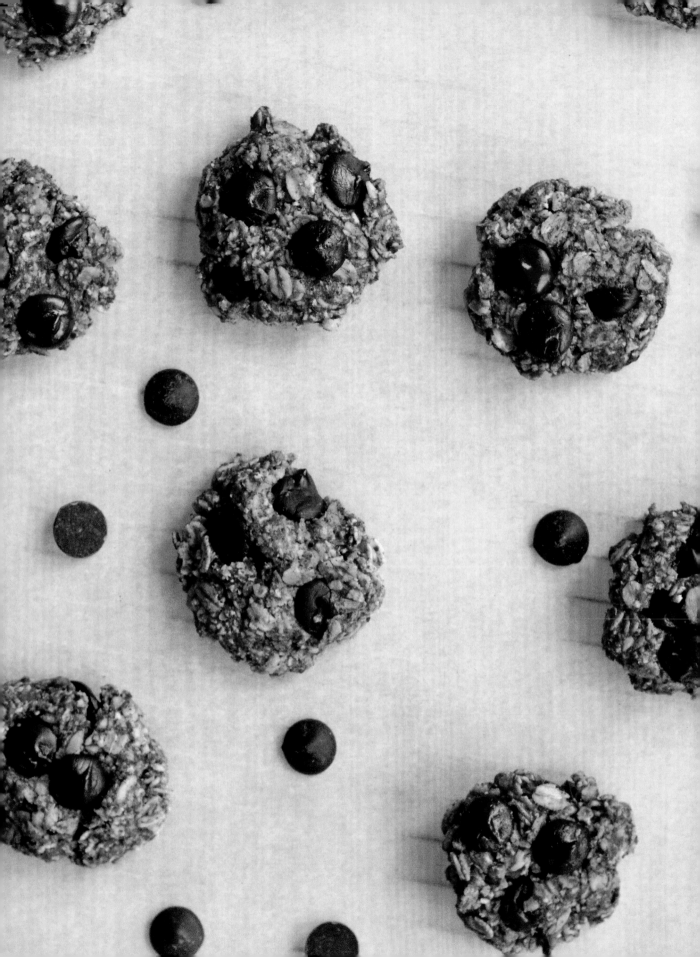

ALMOND BUTTER CHOCOLATE CHIP BREAKFAST COOKIES

MAKES 12 COOKIES   •   **PREP TIME: 5 MINUTES / COOK TIME: 15 MINUTES**

Who doesn't want to start their day with some yummy cookies? These crispy cookies have all the ingredients of a bowl of oatmeal baked into a comforting cookie. Their portability makes them the ideal grab-and-go preworkout breakfast or snack option. Oats are a complex carb, which is slowly digested to provide long-lasting energy during endurance activity. Make a big batch to have a quick, healthy, and satisfying snack throughout the week.

I tablespoon flax meal

3 tablespoons warm water

1½ cups rolled oats

⅓ cup almond butter

¼ cup maple syrup

I teaspoon ground cinnamon

¼ cup dark chocolate chips

Preheat the oven to 350°F. Line a large baking sheet with parchment paper.

In a small bowl, make a flax egg by combining the flax meal and water. Let sit for at least 5 minutes, until the mixture thickens slightly.

In a large bowl, combine the oats, almond butter, maple syrup, cinnamon, and flax egg. Stir until well combined. Add the chocolate chips to the mixture and stir again.

Press the mixture into 2-inch balls and transfer them to the prepared baking sheet. Bake for 15 minutes.

Transfer to a cooling rack and let cool for 10 minutes, then serve warm. Store leftover cookies in a sealed container at room temperature for up to 5 days.

PER SERVING (2 COOKIES): Calories: 270, Fat: 13g, Sat Fat: 3.5g, Sodium: 35mg, Carbohydrates: 34g, Dietary Fiber: 5g, Added Sugar: 11g, Protein: 7g, Vitamin D: 0mcg, Calcium: 84mg, Iron: 2mg, Potassium: 284mg

Fun Facts

All types of oats, including quick-cook, rolled, and steel-cut, have the same nutrition content. The only difference is how the oat is rolled and cut.

RASPBERRY OAT BARS

MAKES 12 SERVINGS • PREP TIME: 5 MINUTES / COOK TIME: 40 MINUTES

This recipe may look like it should be in the dessert chapter, but it's actually the ideal combination of ingredients and nutrients for a preworkout option. The crust and topping are made from healthy carbs, like whole wheat flour, oats, and maple syrup, and a dash of almond butter for nutty flavor that binds it all together. The filling has cooked raspberries, which are inherently sweet and tangy, and a touch of maple syrup and lemon zest. Although a bit more labor intensive than some of the other preworkout recipes, these bars are definitely worth the time in the kitchen.

FOR THE CRUST AND CRUMBLE

2 cups whole wheat flour

1 cup rolled oats

½ cup maple syrup

½ cup almond butter

½ cup vegetable oil

1 teaspoon baking powder

1 teaspoon vanilla extract

½ teaspoon salt

Cooking spray (optional)

FOR THE FILLING

12 ounces raspberries

¼ cup maple syrup

1 teaspoon grated lemon zest

2 teaspoons cornstarch

Preheat the oven to 350°F.

To make the crust and crumble, in a large bowl, combine the flour, oats, maple syrup, almond butter, vegetable oil, baking powder, vanilla, and salt. Stir until combined. The mixture should be crumbly.

Line an 8-inch square baking pan with parchment paper or spray with cooking spray, if using. Spoon half of the oat mixture into the prepared pan and press until it forms a crust. Bake for 10 minutes, then set aside to cool.

Meanwhile, make the filling. In a medium saucepan over medium-high heat, combine the raspberries, maple syrup, lemon zest, and cornstarch. Cook, using a wooden spoon to break down the raspberries, for 10 minutes, until a jam forms.

Spread the jam over the cooled crust. Sprinkle the remaining oat mixture on top and bake for 20 minutes, until the crumble is golden. Set the bars aside and let them cool to the touch. Slice into 12 bars and serve warm. Store leftover bars in a sealed container in the fridge for up to 5 days. Microwave on high power for 20 seconds before eating.

PER SERVING: Calories: 320, Fat: 16g, Sat Fat: 2g, Sodium: 125mg, Carbohydrates: 39g, Dietary Fiber: 6g, Added Sugar: 12g, Protein: 6g, Vitamin D: 0mcg, Calcium: 124mg, Iron: 2mg, Potassium: 265mg

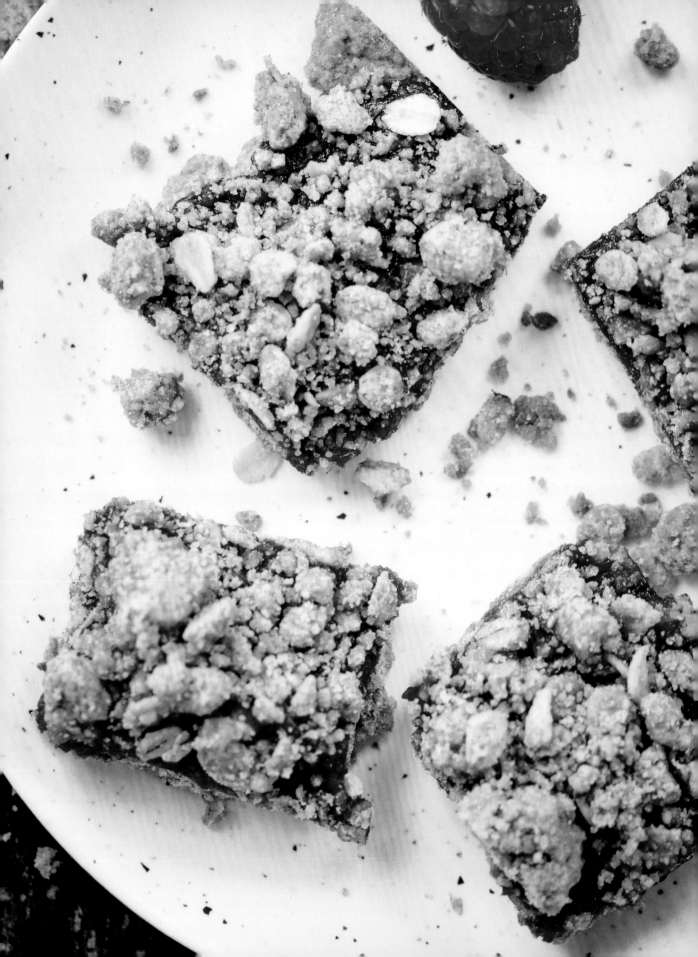

BLUEBERRY AND CINNAMON APPLE SMOOTHIE

MAKES 2 SERVINGS • PREP TIME: 5 MINUTES

You may not think blueberries and apples go together, but trust me that this flavor combination just works. With a hint of cinnamon, this smoothie tastes like fall and summer all in one glass. The sweetness from the apples and blueberries stands out, and you may not even need the honey or maple syrup. Feel free to use a plain nondairy yogurt instead of Greek yogurt, but be aware that plant-based yogurts are usually much lower in protein. Either way, this smoothie is a simple preworkout snack that offers plenty of quick-acting carbs for energy.

1 Gala apple or other red apple, sliced

1 cup frozen blueberries

1 cup plain nonfat Greek yogurt or nondairy yogurt

½ cup water

1 teaspoon ground cinnamon

1 teaspoon honey or maple syrup (optional)

In a blender, combine the apple, blueberries, yogurt, water, cinnamon, and honey, if using. Blend until smooth.

PER SERVING: Calories: 170, Fat: 1.5g, Sat Fat: 0g, Sodium: 45mg, Carbohydrates: 29g, Dietary Fiber: 5g, Added Sugar: 0g, Protein: 13g, Vitamin D: 0mcg, Calcium: 167mg, Iron: 1mg, Potassium: 322mg

Fun Facts

One of the biggest struggles among endurance athletes is tummy troubles. Eating the wrong thing before or during a workout can cause GI issues that interfere with your ability to perform. To prevent stomach issues, experiment with different fueling routines to find one that causes the fewest number of issues.

CANDIED MAPLE GINGER WALNUTS

MAKES 8 SERVINGS • PREP TIME: 5 MINUTES / COOK TIME: 20 MINUTES

These baked walnuts have so much flavor in one little bite. The sweetness from the maple syrup pairs nicely with the kick from the ginger, all topped off with a hint of salt. Plus, the healthy omega-3s in walnuts have been linked to heart and brain health, as well as hunger control. Incorporating healthy fats into snacks helps satisfy your appetite between meals. Add this snack to your recovery routine for some much-needed protein and fat.

2 cups chopped unsalted walnuts

¼ cup maple syrup

1 teaspoon ground ginger

¼ teaspoon salt

Preheat the oven to 325°F. Line a large baking sheet with parchment paper.

In a large bowl, combine the walnuts, maple syrup, ginger, and salt. Stir until well combined.

Spread the walnuts on the prepared baking sheet and bake for 20 minutes or until caramelized. Serve warm. Store leftover walnuts in a sealed container at room temperature for up to 5 days.

PER SERVING: Calories: 180, Fat: 15g, Sat Fat: 1.5g, Sodium: 75mg, Carbohydrates: 10g, Dietary Fiber: 2g, Added Sugar: 6g, Protein: 4g, Vitamin D: 0mcg, Calcium: 26mg, Iron: 1mg, Potassium: 24mg

Fun Facts

Newer research suggests that eating 1.5 ounces of walnuts per day may positively impact the gut microbiome, otherwise known as the "good bacteria" in the gut. These little critters promote overall immune health and may play a role in brain health.

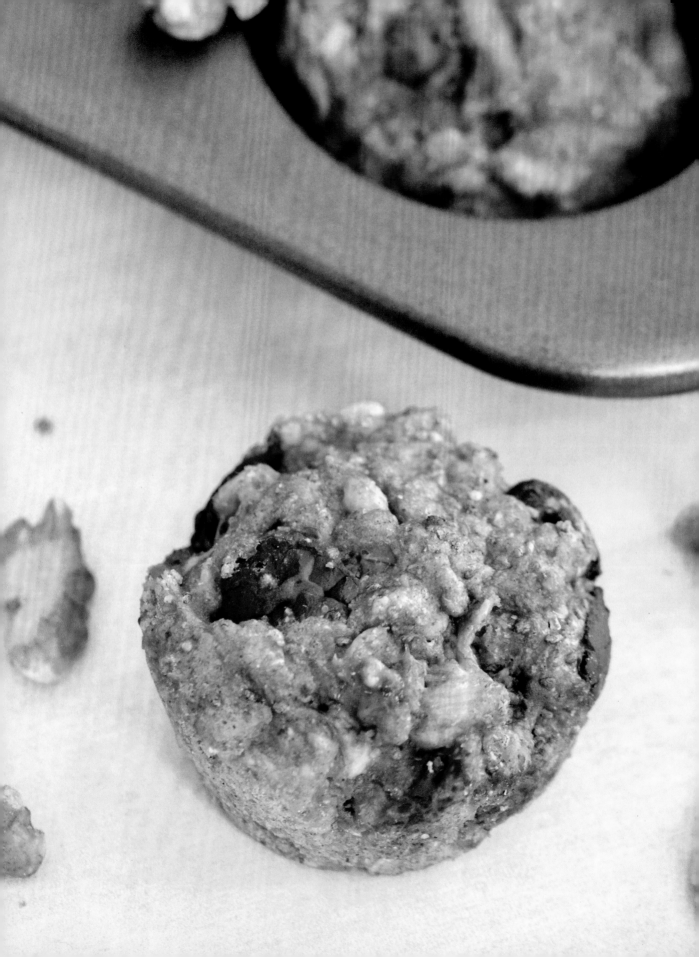

WHOLE WHEAT BANANA NUT MUFFINS

MAKES 12 MUFFINS • **PREP TIME: 10 MINUTES / COOK TIME: 20 MINUTES**

These muffins are packed with whole grain goodness, and they are much healthier than any store-bought variety. Sweetened by the banana, these muffins will satisfy your sweet tooth and fill you up before a workout. They are hearty, dense, and filling, and they are travel friendly for busy mornings. As an added bonus, bananas are packed with potassium, an important mineral that plays a role in hydration and blood flow.

Cooking spray (optional)

2 tablespoons chia seeds

¼ cup water

2 ripe bananas, mashed

½ cup unsweetened almond milk

⅓ cup maple syrup

¼ cup neutral oil (canola, vegetable, or grapeseed)

1 teaspoon vanilla extract

1½ cups whole wheat flour

¼ cup rolled oats

2 teaspoons ground cinnamon

1 teaspoon baking powder

¼ teaspoon salt

¼ cup chopped unsalted walnuts

¼ cup semisweet chocolate chips (optional)

Preheat the oven to 350°F. Line 12 standard muffin cups with silicone or paper liners, or spray well with cooking spray, if using.

In a large bowl, combine the chia seeds and water. Mix well and let stand for 5 minutes, or until the mixture becomes thick. Add the mashed bananas, almond milk, maple syrup, neutral oil, and vanilla. Whisk together until well combined.

In a separate large bowl, combine the whole wheat flour, oats, cinnamon, baking powder, and salt. Mix well.

Add the banana mixture to the flour mixture and stir until combined. Add the walnuts and chocolate chips, if using, and stir to combine.

Fill each prepared muffin cup three-quarters full with batter. Bake for 20 minutes, or until a toothpick inserted into the center of a muffin comes out clean. Serve warm. Store leftover muffins in a sealed container at room temperature for up to 3 days or in the fridge for up to 7 days. If desired, microwave for 30 seconds before eating.

PER SERVING (2 MUFFINS): Calories: 340, Fat: 15g, Sat Fat: 2g, Sodium: 130mg, Carbohydrates: 49g, Dietary Fiber: 7g, Added Sugar: 11g, Protein: 7g, Vitamin D: 0mcg, Calcium: 210mg, Iron: 2mg, Potassium: 319mg

KEY LIME QUICK BREAD

MAKES 8 SERVINGS • **PREP TIME: 10 MINUTES / COOK TIME: 45 MINUTES**

My husband is a huge fan of anything lime flavored, which inspired me to create this quick bread. You may be surprised to find seltzer among the ingredients, but it acts as a plant-based egg replacement. Although it sounds crazy, it absolutely works to bind the bread together. The result is a light and fluffy bread with a tangy lime flavor. Have a slice of this moist bread before an early morning workout or for a midafternoon sweet treat.

Cooking spray

1½ cups whole wheat flour

1 cup all-purpose flour

1 teaspoon baking powder

½ teaspoon baking soda

Pinch salt

⅔ cup maple syrup

⅔ cup unsweetened almond milk or plant milk of choice

½ cup vegetable oil

½ cup plain seltzer

Grated zest of 2 limes

⅓ cup fresh lime juice

Preheat the oven to 350°F. Spray a 9 × 5-inch loaf pan with cooking spray.

In a large bowl, combine the whole wheat flour, all-purpose flour, baking powder, baking soda, and salt. Mix well.

In a separate large bowl, combine the maple syrup, almond milk, vegetable oil, seltzer, lime zest, and lime juice. Whisk until well combined.

Add the seltzer mixture to the flour mixture and stir until combined.

Pour the batter into the prepared pan and bake for 45 minutes, or until a toothpick inserted into the center comes out clean. Serve warm. Garnish with some lime zest. Store leftover bread in a sealed container at room temperature for up to 3 days.

PER SERVING: Calories: 330, Fat: 15g, Sat Fat: 2g, Sodium: 170mg, Carbohydrates: 48g, Dietary Fiber: 3g, Added Sugar: 16g, Protein: 5g, Vitamin D: 0mcg, Calcium: 152mg, Iron: 1mg, Potassium: 164mg

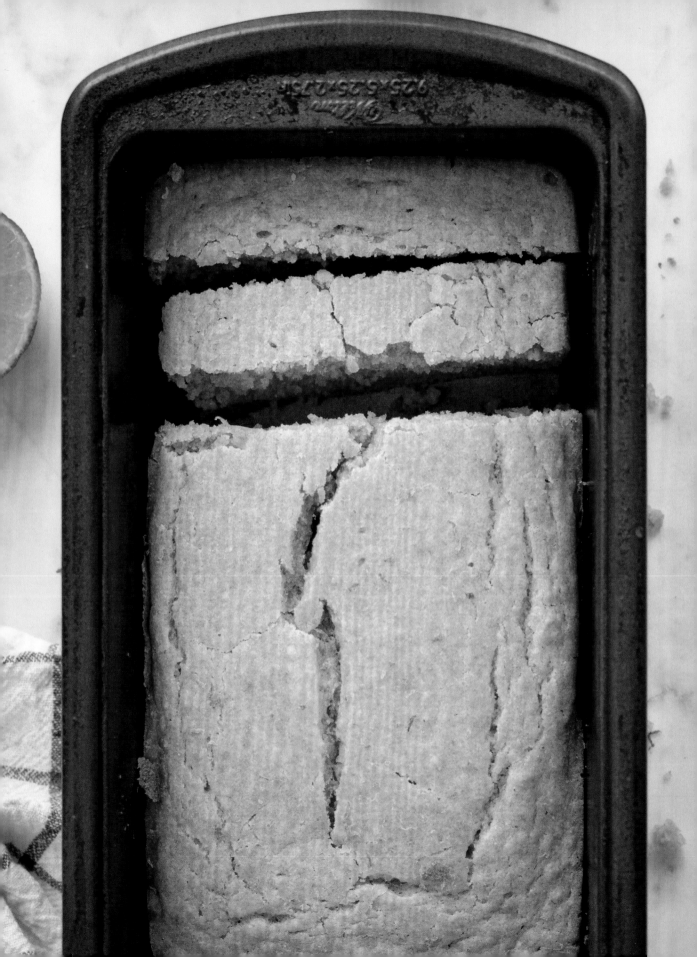

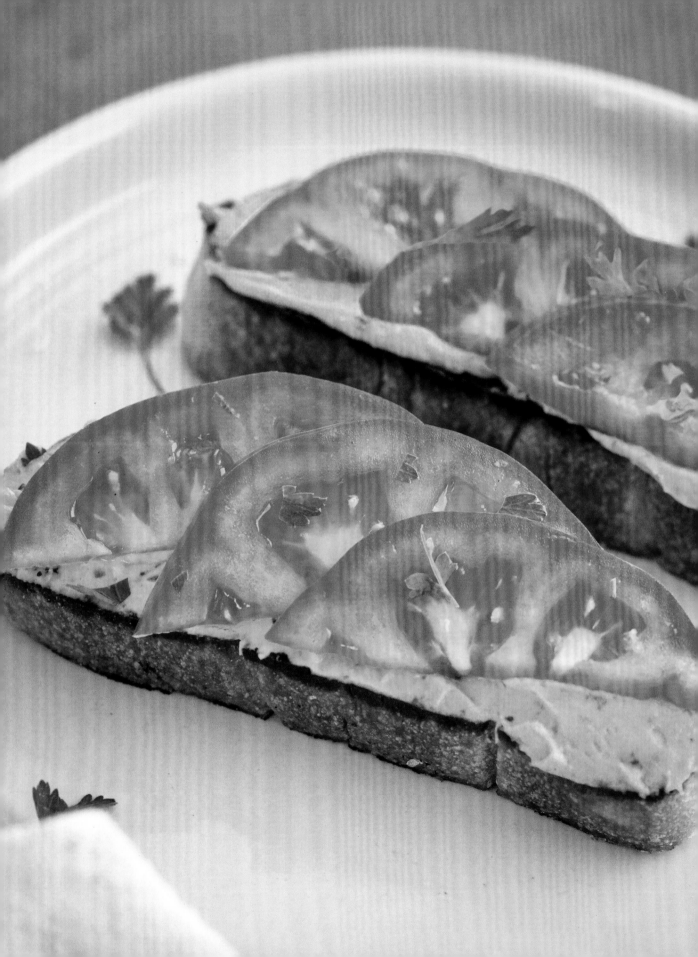

AVOCADO YOGURT CIABATTA BREAD

MAKES 4 SERVINGS • **PREP TIME: 10 MINUTES / COOK TIME: 10 MINUTES**

My husband asks for this "breakfast bread" on special occasions because it's so darn delicious. And the best part is that it's really easy to make, even though it looks like a fancy (and expensive) brunch item. Top toasted ciabatta bread with a protein- and healthy fat–packed avocado yogurt spread. Then finish it off with ripe tomato slices and coarse sea salt for a filling, vibrant, and yummy breakfast toast.

8 slices ciabatta bread

2 tablespoons extra-virgin olive oil

1 teaspoon paprika

1 avocado, pitted and peeled

¼ cup plain nonfat Greek yogurt or nondairy yogurt

2 tablespoons fresh cilantro or flat-leaf parsley leaves

1 tablespoon fresh lime juice

¼ teaspoon salt

1 tomato, sliced

Coarse salt

Place the bread slices on a cutting board. Drizzle the olive oil and sprinkle the paprika evenly over the bread.

Heat a large sauté pan over medium-high heat. Place the pieces of bread in the pan, olive oil side down. Cook for 5 minutes, then flip and cook for 1 to 2 minutes longer, until each side begins to brown.

While the bread cooks, place the avocado, yogurt, cilantro, lime juice, and salt in a food processor and process until smooth.

Remove the bread from the pan and use a knife to slather on the avocado yogurt, then top with the tomato slices. Sprinkle coarse sea salt on each piece of bread and serve warm.

PER SERVING: Calories: 300, Fat: 14g, Sat Fat: 2g, Sodium: 540mg, Carbohydrates: 36g, Dietary Fiber: 3g, Added Sugar: 0g, Protein: 10g, Vitamin D: 0mcg, Calcium: 105mg, Iron: 3mg, Potassium: 376mg

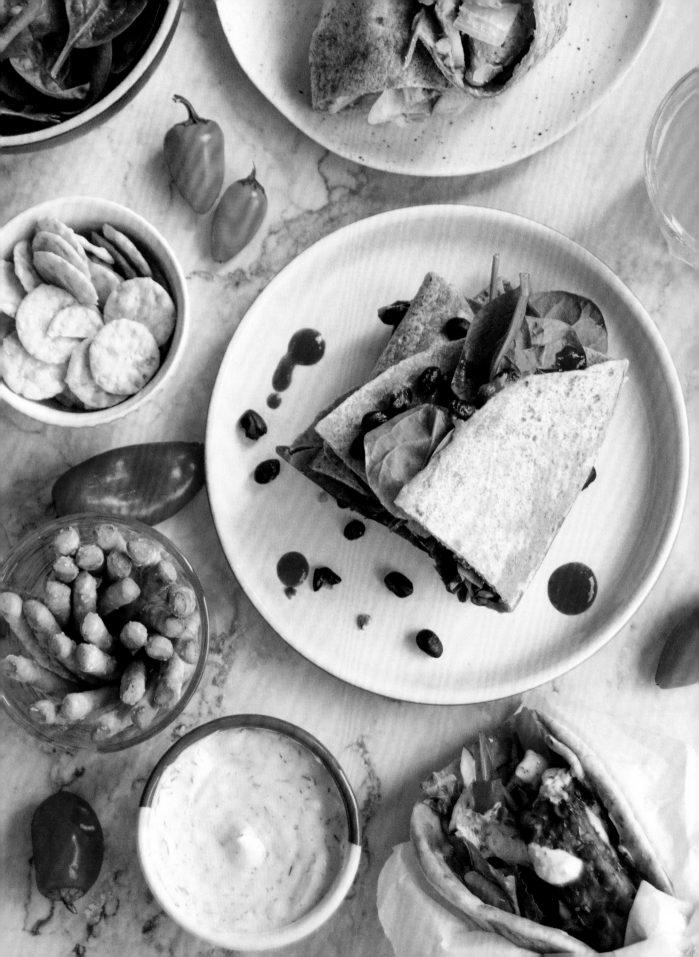

CHAPTER 4

LUNCHES TO NOURISH AN EVENING WORKOUT

If you exercise at night, chances are you've gone into a workout hungry, drained, and unmotivated. Believe it or not, fueling for a nighttime workout starts at lunch. Eating a well-balanced meal that sticks with you throughout the afternoon helps propel you into any type of evening workout, whether it's an intense track session or a spin class. These recipes have a healthy balance of colorful veggies, plant-based proteins, and good fats to keep energy levels high for an evening workout.

KALE, CITRUS, AND NUT SALAD

MAKES 4 SERVINGS • PREP TIME: 10 MINUTES

All you need are three simple ingredients to make this winter salad. Dark kale combined with juicy ruby red grapefruit and salty pistachios, topped with a citrusy dressing, make an upscale salad that can accompany any other lunch item in this chapter. Or add some protein, such as quinoa, chickpeas, or roasted tofu, to make this a balanced and light lunch.

FOR THE DRESSING
¼ cup extra-virgin olive oil

2 tablespoons fresh orange juice

1 tablespoon red wine vinegar

½ tablespoon honey or maple syrup

Salt

FOR THE SALAD
8 cups chopped stemmed kale

4 ruby red grapefruit, peeled and diced

¼ cup shelled salted pistachios

To make the dressing, in a small bowl, whisk together the olive oil, orange juice, vinegar, and honey. Season to taste with salt.

To make the salad, in a large bowl, combine the kale, grapefruit, and pistachios. Pour the dressing on top and toss well. Store leftover salad and dressing in separate sealed containers in the fridge for up to 5 days.

PER SERVING: Calories: 310, Fat: 17g, Sat Fat: 2.5g, Sodium: 200mg, Carbohydrates: 38g, Dietary Fiber: 6g, Added Sugar: 2g, Protein: 5g, Vitamin D: 0mcg, Calcium: 99mg, Iron: 1mg, Potassium: 253mg

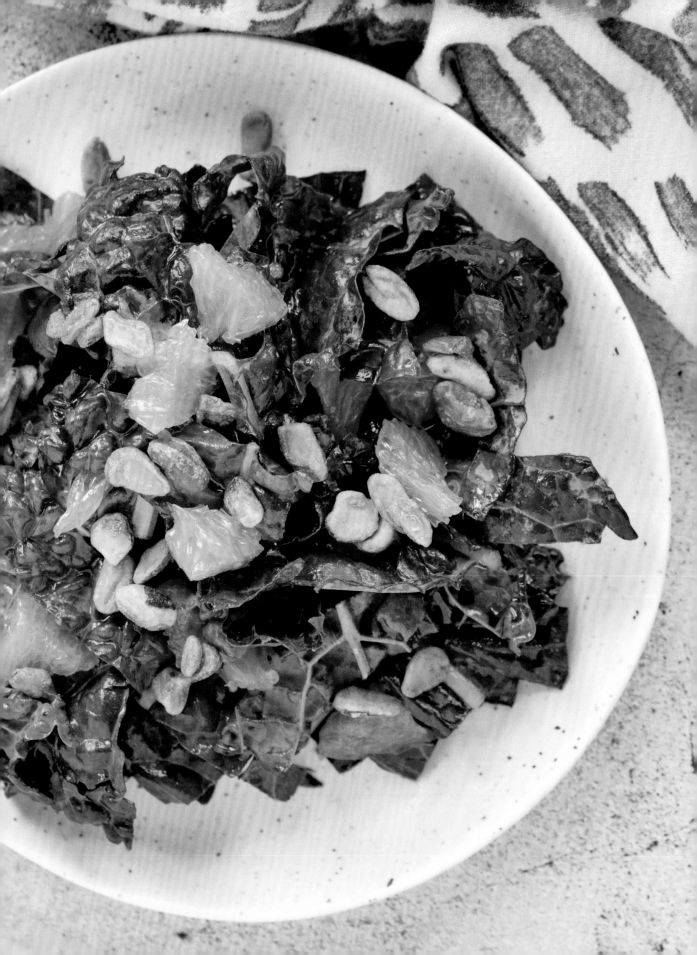

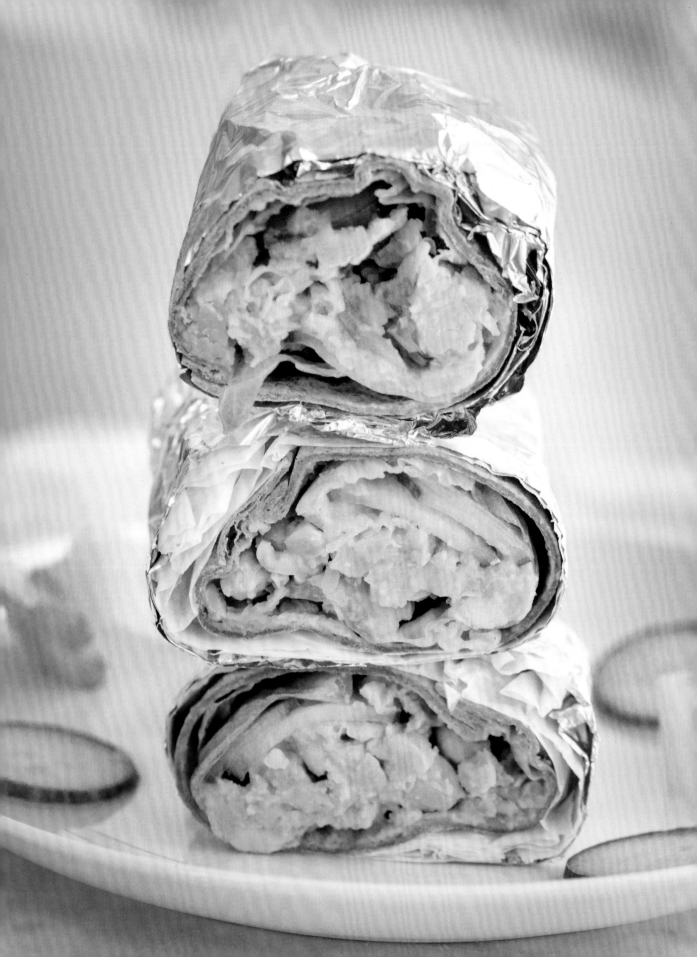

CHICKPEA AVOCADO SMASH WRAP

MAKES 4 SERVINGS • **PREP TIME: 10 MINUTES**

This is my go-to lunch, and I bring it just about anywhere: long hikes, a day in the park, or even a busy day of errands. The base is made with three simple ingredients—chickpeas, avocado, and lemon juice—which creates a hearty and flavorful start of a sandwich. Then add some sliced cucumbers and lettuce for crunch in a hearty whole wheat wrap. These simple ingredients combined provide big flavor, as well as plenty of plant-based protein.

2 cans (15.5 oz) chickpeas, drained and rinsed

1 avocado, pitted and peeled

¼ cup fresh lemon juice

½ teaspoon salt

Freshly ground black pepper

4 whole wheat wraps, large (10 inches)

1 small cucumber, thinly sliced

2 cups coarsely chopped butter lettuce or romaine lettuce

In a large bowl, combine the chickpeas, avocado, lemon juice, and salt. Season to taste with black pepper. Use a fork or potato masher to mash everything together until you have a chunky consistency.

Lay the wraps on a work surface and top each with cucumber, lettuce, and 1 cup of smashed chickpeas. Roll up into wraps. Store leftover wraps in a sealed container in the fridge for up to 3 days. (The avocado may brown, but it is still safe to eat.)

PER SERVING: Calories: 520, Fat: 16g, Sat Fat: 3.5g, Sodium: 880mg, Carbohydrates: 78g, Dietary Fiber: 16g, Added Sugar: 0g, Protein: 22g, Vitamin D: 0mcg, Calcium: 231mg, Iron: 5mg, Potassium: 752mg

RAINBOW VEGGIE SANDWICH

MAKES 2 SERVINGS • **PREP TIME: 10 MINUTES**

Plant-based sandwiches don't need to be boring old lettuce, tomato, and hummus. As a matter of fact, there is a sandwich shop in New York City that makes a delicious and nutritious veggie sandwich with all the fixings, which is the inspiration for my version. For this sandwich, you'll whip up a homemade honey-mustard dressing, then pile colorful veggies onto whole wheat bread. You'll need to open wide to take a big bite of all these yummy veggies together.

2 tablespoons extra-virgin olive oil

1 tablespoon red wine vinegar

1 tablespoon honey

1 tablespoon Dijon mustard

Salt

4 slices whole wheat bread

½ cup coarsely chopped romaine lettuce

1 tomato, sliced

½ cup shredded red cabbage

½ small cucumber, thinly sliced

½ cup shredded carrots

1 avocado, pitted, peeled, and sliced

½ cup alfalfa sprouts

In a small bowl, make the dressing by whisking together the olive oil, vinegar, honey, and mustard. Season to taste with salt.

Lay out two pieces of bread and drizzle each side with about half of the dressing. Layer the bread with half of the remaining ingredients: romaine lettuce, tomato, cabbage, cucumber, carrots, avocado, and alfalfa sprouts. Top with a second slice of bread. Repeat this step for the second sandwich.

Slice and serve right away.

PER SERVING: Calories: 440, Fat: 27g, Sat Fat: 3.5g, Sodium: 690mg, Carbohydrates: 45g, Dietary Fiber: 11g, Added Sugar: 11g, Protein: 7g, Vitamin D: 0mcg, Calcium: 100mg, Iron: 3mg, Potassium: 751mg

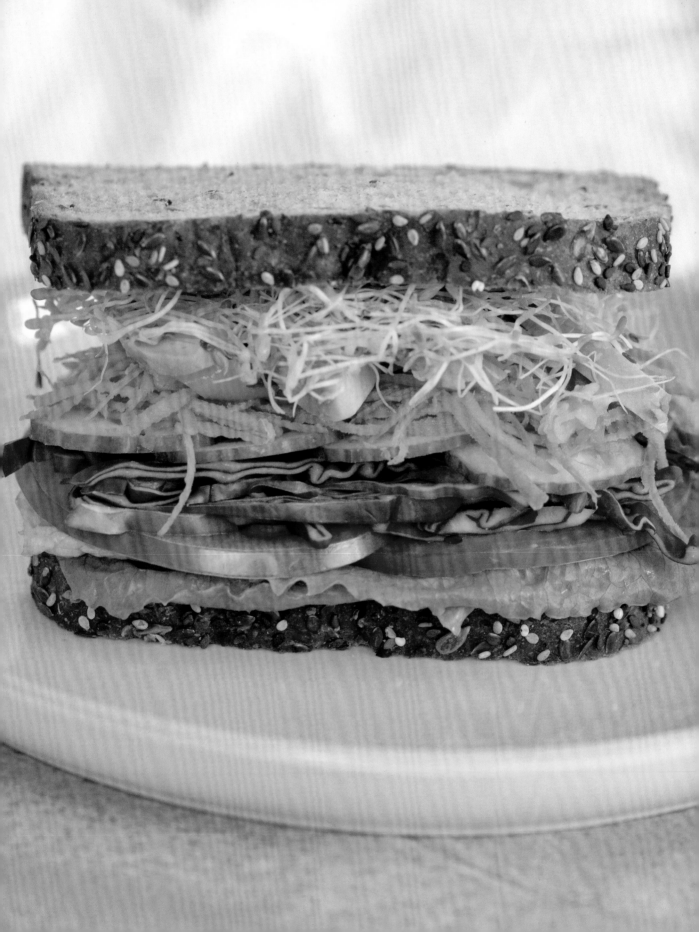

TEMPEH GYRO WITH TOFU TZATZIKI SAUCE

MAKES 4 SERVINGS • **PREP TIME: 10 MINUTES / COOK TIME: 15 MINUTES**

A gyro is a Greek sandwich made with marinated meat stuffed in pita bread, served with a yogurt tzatziki sauce. This plant-based version uses marinated tempeh to replace the meat and silken tofu as a stand-in for yogurt. The end result is just as filling and delicious as the traditional sandwich. The tempeh has plenty of protein and a "meaty" taste that is coated with flavorful spices and herbs. It's finished with a creamy tzatziki sauce and wrapped in a flatbread with all the best sandwich fixings.

FOR THE TEMPEH

½ cup diced white onion

4 cloves garlic, minced

¼ cup low-sodium soy sauce

½ cup water

1 teaspoon dried oregano

½ teaspoon dried rosemary

½ teaspoon freshly ground black pepper

2 tablespoons extra-virgin olive oil

1 package (16 oz) tempeh

FOR THE TZATZIKI SAUCE

8 ounces silken tofu

2 tablespoons fresh lemon juice

2 cloves garlic

1 tablespoon fresh dill leaves

¼ teaspoon salt

½ cup chopped cucumber

To make the tempeh, in a small bowl, mix together the onion, garlic, soy sauce, water, oregano, rosemary, and black pepper. Set aside.

Heat a large sauté pan over medium heat, then pour in the olive oil and add the tempeh. Sauté for 2 minutes on each side, until golden brown.

Add the soy sauce mixture, cover, reduce the heat to low, and simmer for 10 minutes, until all the liquid is absorbed.

Meanwhile, make the tzatziki sauce. In a food processor, combine the tofu, lemon juice, garlic, dill, and salt. Process until smooth. Remove the mixture from the food processor and stir in the cucumbers.

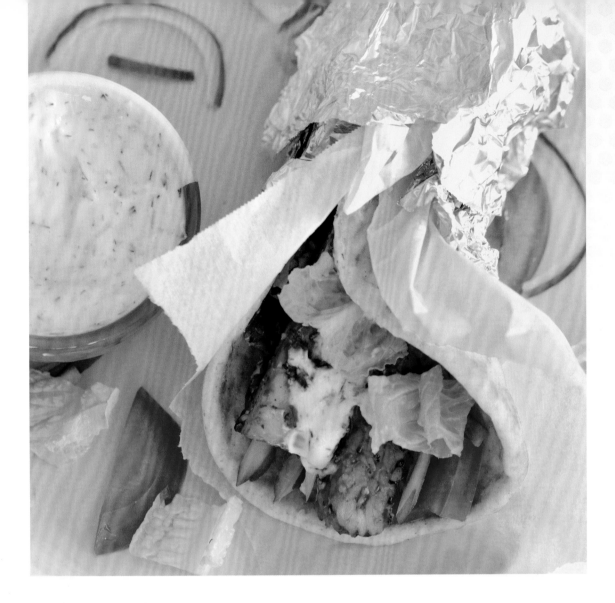

FOR THE SANDWICHES

4 flatbreads

2 cups chopped romaine
lettuce

2 tomatoes, sliced

½ red onion, sliced (⅓ cup)

To make the sandwiches, top each flatbread with
tempeh, tzatziki sauce, lettuce, tomato, and onion. Serve
immediately or store each component in separate
containers in the fridge for up to 5 days. Microwave and
assemble the sandwiches when ready to eat.

PER SERVING: Calories: 400, Fat: 22g, Sat Fat: 4g, Sodium: 990mg, Carbohydrates: 28g,
Dietary Fiber: 2g, Added Sugar: 1g, Protein: 30g, Vitamin D: 0mcg, Calcium: 235mg, Iron:
5mg, Potassium: 835mg

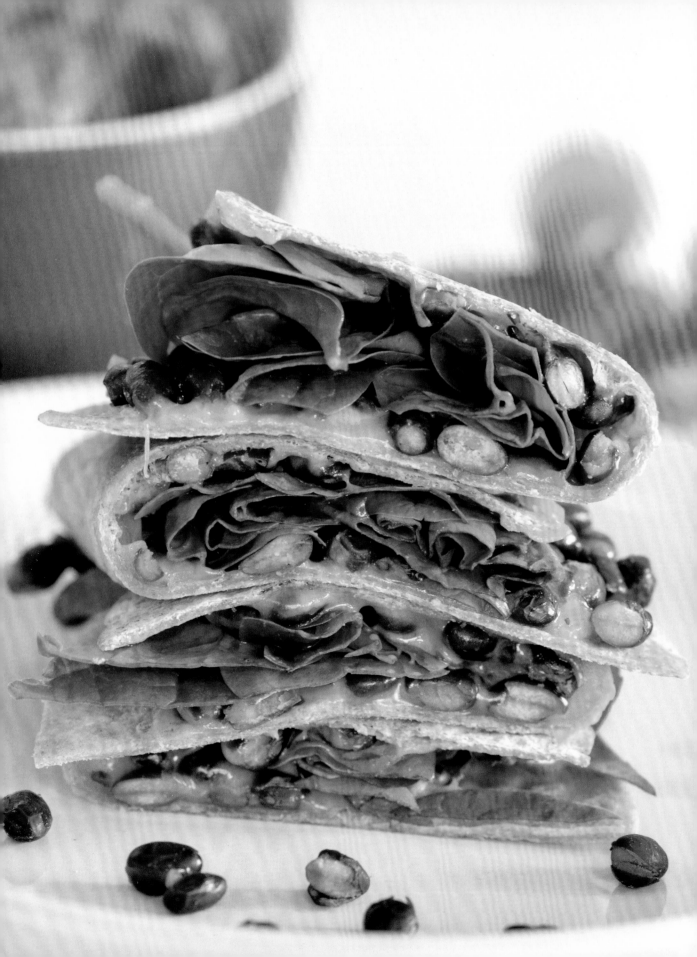

BLACK BEAN QUESADILLAS

MAKES 2 SERVINGS • PREP TIME: 5 MINUTES / COOK TIME: 10 MINUTES PER QUESADILLA

This is my go-to lunch when I'm short on time. It takes just 15 minutes to make, and it's yummy, comforting, and full of flavor. And you only need a few simple ingredients to throw it all together. Black beans and cheese serve as the base of this quesadilla, with a heaping handful of spinach and a drizzle of sriracha. It may sound simple (and it is), but it's also nourishing and tasty with a hint of spiciness.

2 whole wheat tortillas, large (10 inches)

½ cup shredded Cheddar cheese (see tip)

1 cup drained and rinsed black beans

Cooking spray

2 cups packed spinach

2 teaspoons sriracha

Place 1 tortilla flat on a plate or cutting board. Sprinkle ¼ cup of cheese and ½ cup of black beans on one side of the tortilla. Fold the tortilla in half. You may have to hold it shut until you put it in the pan.

Heat a large frying pan over medium heat. Coat with cooking spray. Add the tortilla to the pan and cook for 3 to 5 minutes on one side. Flip and cook on the other side for 3 to 5 minutes longer, until both sides are golden brown.

Remove the quesadilla from the pan and open it slightly to place 1 cup of spinach and 1 teaspoon of sriracha inside.

Repeat all steps to make the second quesadilla. Serve immediately.

PER SERVING: Calories: 350, Fat: 13g, Sat Fat: 7g, Sodium: 560mg, Carbohydrates: 42g, Dietary Fiber: 11g, Added Sugar: 1g, Protein: 18g, Vitamin D: 0mcg, Calcium: 282mg, Iron: 4mg, Potassium: 653mg

Vegan Tip: Replace the Cheddar with vegan cheddar or 2 tablespoons of hummus.

EDAMAME RICE BOWL WITH MISO DRESSING

MAKES 4 SERVINGS • **PREP TIME: 15 MINUTES**

Edamame is a truly underrated plant-based protein that I always keep in my freezer. This sushi staple has 10 grams of protein in a ½-cup serving, and it's also full of fiber (24 percent of the daily value) to keep you full throughout the afternoon. This simple bowl combines crunchy veggies, such as carrots, cabbage, and cucumber, with rice, edamame, and avocado all under a sweet and salty miso dressing. Since the rice tends to absorb the flavors of the dressing the longer it sits, I encourage you to make a big batch of this and nosh on it for lunch all week.

FOR THE RICE BOWL

2 cups cooked brown rice

2 cups cooked edamame

1 cup shredded carrots

1 cup shredded red cabbage

2 avocados, pitted, peeled, and chopped

1 small cucumber, thinly sliced

Salt

FOR THE DRESSING

2 tablespoons white, light, or yellow miso paste

2 tablespoons sesame oil

2 tablespoons rice vinegar

1 tablespoon low-sodium soy sauce

2 teaspoons maple syrup

½ teaspoon grated fresh ginger

To make the rice bowl, in a large bowl, combine the rice, edamame, carrots, red cabbage, avocados, and cucumber. Season to taste with salt.

To make the dressing, in a small bowl, whisk together the miso paste, sesame oil, vinegar, soy sauce, maple syrup, and ginger.

Pour the dressing over the rice mixture. Serve warm or store in sealed containers in the fridge for up to 5 days.

PER SERVING: Calories: 620, Fat: 24g, Sat Fat: 3g, Sodium: 770mg, Carbohydrates: 89g, Dietary Fiber: 12g, Added Sugar: 2g, Protein: 18g, Vitamin D: 0mcg, Calcium: 87mg, Iron: 4mg, Potassium: 1,042mg

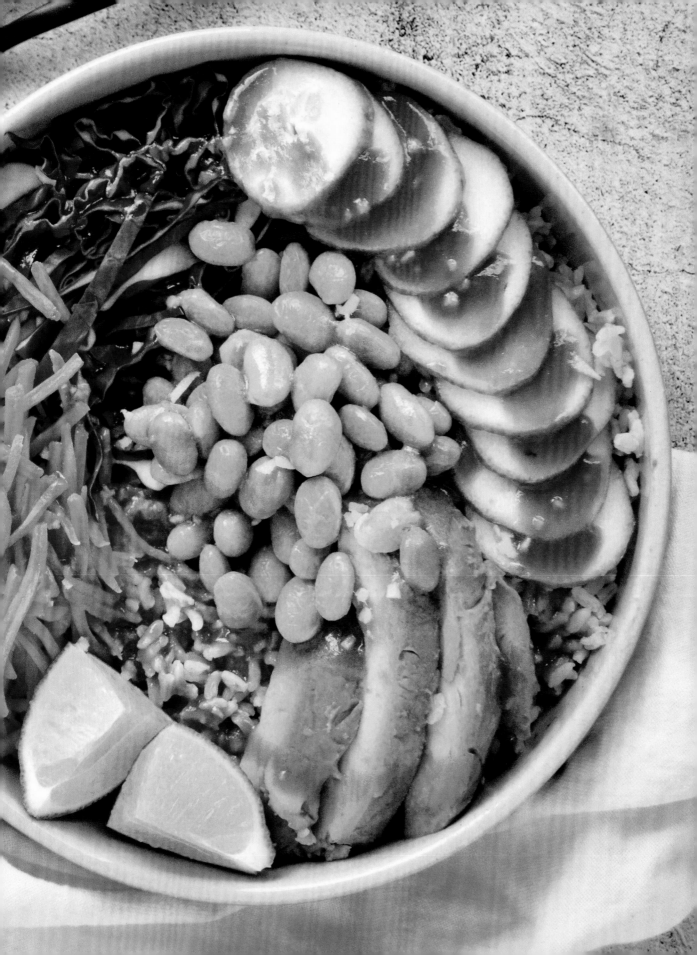

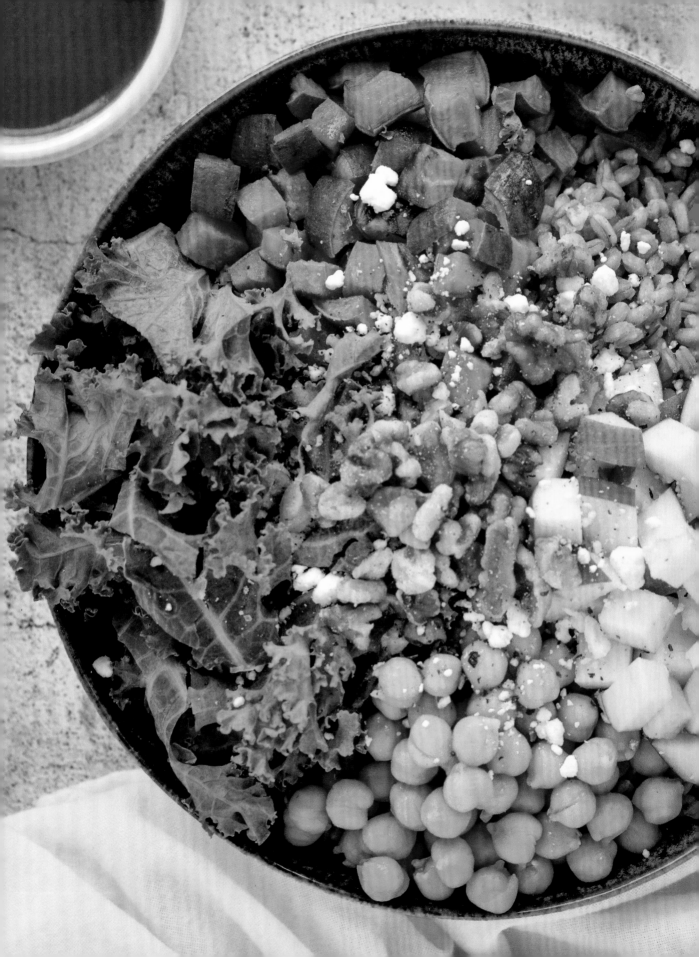

FALL SWEET POTATO, APPLE, KALE, AND FARRO BOWL

MAKES 6 SERVINGS • **PREP TIME: 10 MINUTES / COOK TIME: 40 MINUTES**

Fall is one of my favorite seasons not only because of the beautiful weather and foliage but also the produce. And this recipe is fall in a bowl, with sweet potatoes, apples, and kale over a bowl of whole grain goodness. Farro is an ancient grain that is used in many Italian dishes. It's slightly chewy with a nutty taste and hearty texture. Opt for the quick-cooking farro varieties to cut the cooking time down to just 10 minutes (as opposed to 45 minutes). The bowl is topped off with some chickpeas, goat cheese, and walnuts for extra protein.

FOR THE FARRO BOWL
- 2 cups quick-cooking (pearled) farro
- 2 sweet potatoes, cubed (about 4 cups)
- 1 tablespoon extra-virgin olive oil
- ¼ teaspoon salt
- 2 apples, chopped
- 2 cups chopped stemmed kale
- 2 cups drained and rinsed chickpeas
- ½ cup goat cheese or vegan goat cheese
- ¼ cup chopped unsalted walnuts

FOR THE DRESSING
- ¼ cup extra-virgin olive oil
- 2 tablespoons balsamic vinegar
- 1 tablespoon Dijon mustard
- 1 tablespoon maple syrup
- ¼ teaspoon salt

Preheat the oven to 375°F. Line a large baking sheet with aluminum foil.

To make the farro bowl, cook the farro according to package directions, usually about 10 minutes. While the farro cooks, place the sweet potatoes, olive oil, and salt in a small bowl, stirring to combine. Transfer them to the prepared baking sheet, spreading them out in an even layer. Roast for 30 minutes, until the sweet potatoes begins to caramelize.

In a large bowl, combine the apples, kale, chickpeas, goat cheese, and walnuts. Add the cooked farro and sweet potatoes, tossing to combine.

To make the dressing, in a small bowl, whisk together the olive oil, vinegar, mustard, maple syrup, and salt.

Divide the farro mixture into bowls and top with dressing when ready to serve. Serve warm. Store leftover farro bowl and dressing in separate sealed containers in the fridge for up to 5 days.

PER SERVING: Calories: 560, Fat: 20g, Sat Fat: 3.5g, Sodium: 430mg, Carbohydrates: 85g, Dietary Fiber: 14g, Added Sugar: 2g, Protein: 14g, Vitamin D: 0mcg, Calcium: 108mg, Iron: 3mg, Potassium: 716mg

TACO SALAD WITH SRIRACHA RANCH DRESSING

MAKES 4 SERVINGS • PREP TIME: 15 MINUTES / COOK TIME: 20 MINUTES

Bring the joy of sizzling fajitas to your lunch bowl and top it off with a spicy sriracha ranch dressing. This recipe has all of the plant-based fajita foods you know and love, like peppers, onions, romaine lettuce, and cheese, with some protein, like quinoa and black beans. It's topped off with a spicy yogurt sriracha ranch dressing that is so easy to make and will make your taste buds happy. Feel free to skip the cheese and use a plant-based yogurt for a completely vegan dish.

FOR THE TACO SALAD

1 cup quinoa

2 tablespoons extra-virgin olive oil

2 green bell peppers, thinly sliced

1 white onion, thinly sliced (½ cup)

¼ teaspoon salt

2 cups drained and rinsed black beans

4 cups chopped romaine lettuce

2 ounces corn tortilla chips (about 20 chips)

¼ cup shredded Cheddar cheese or vegan cheddar

FOR THE DRESSING

½ cup plain nonfat Greek yogurt or nondairy yogurt

1 tablespoon sriracha

¾ teaspoon garlic powder

1½ teaspoons fresh lemon juice

1 teaspoon dried chives

¼ teaspoon salt

2 tablespoons water

To make the taco salad, cook the quinoa according to package directions, usually 10 to 12 minutes. While the quinoa cooks, heat a large frying pan over medium-high heat. Add the olive oil, bell peppers, onion, and salt. Cook, stirring occasionally, for 10 minutes, until the peppers and onion are soft

Transfer the quinoa and onion-pepper mixture to a large bowl. Add the beans, romaine lettuce, and Cheddar cheese, tossing to combine. Add tortilla chips on the side.

To make the dressing, in a small bowl, combine the yogurt, sriracha, garlic powder, lemon juice, chives, salt, and water. Stir until combined.

Divide the quinoa mixture among bowls and top with dressing when ready to serve. Serve warm. Store leftover salad and dressing in separate sealed containers in the fridge for up to 5 days.

PER SERVING: Calories: 480, Fat: 15g, Sat Fat: 3g, Sodium: 690mg, Carbohydrates: 66g, Dietary Fiber: 12g, Added Sugar: 0g, Protein: 21g, Vitamin D: 0mcg, Calcium: 178mg, Iron: 5mg, Potassium: 746mg

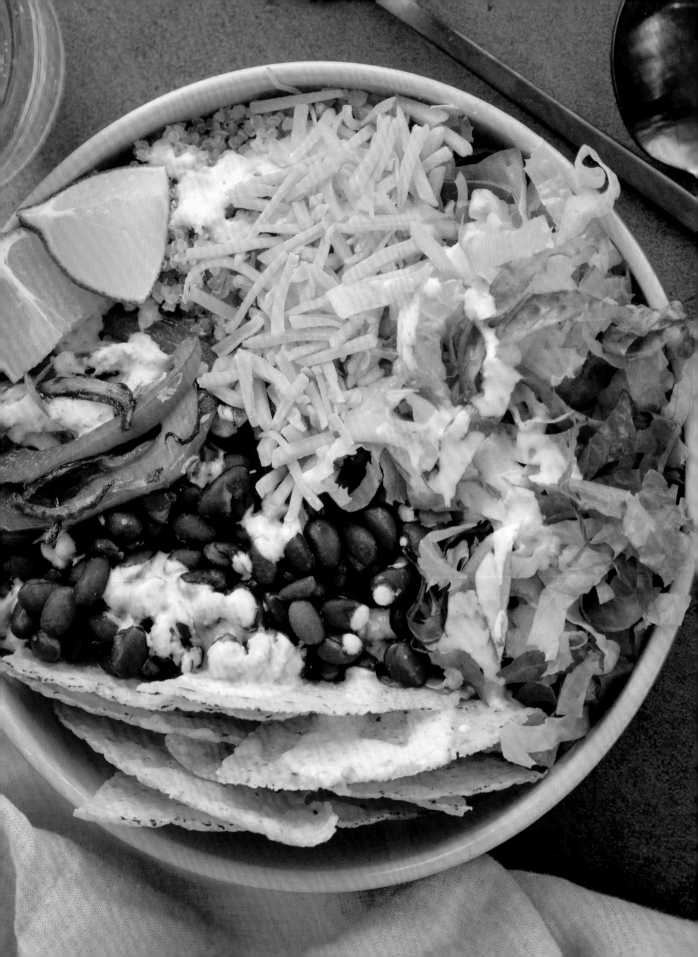

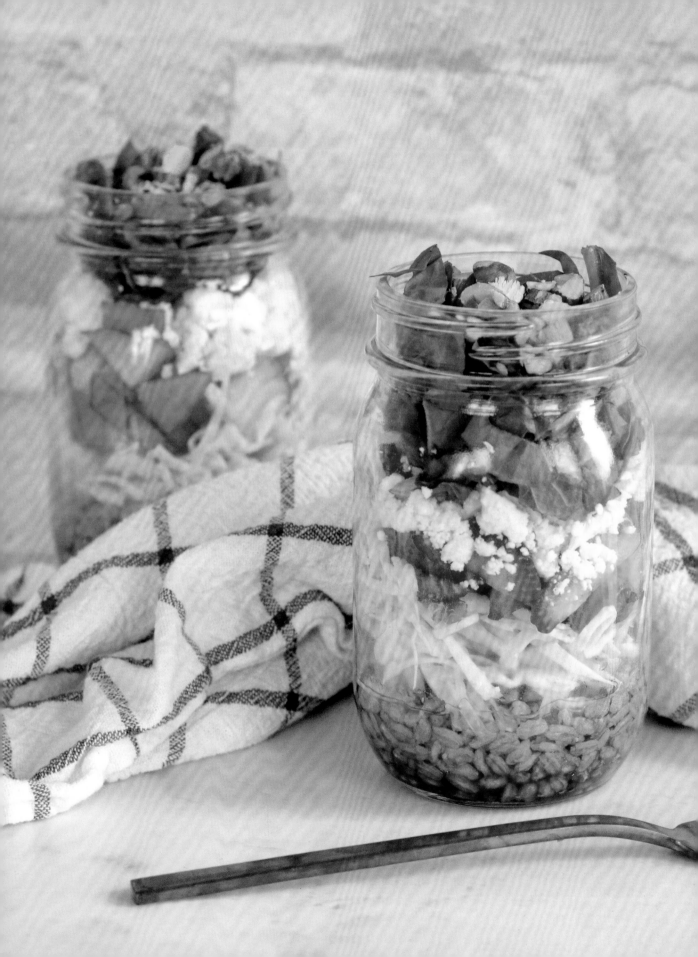

MASON JAR FARRO SALAD

MAKES 4 SERVINGS • **PREP TIME: 15 MINUTES / COOK TIME: 10 MINUTES**

This convenient lunch is built in layers so that you can easily carry it with you without making a mess or ending up with soggy lettuce. It starts with the dressing on the bottom, followed by grains, hearty veggies, and seasonal fruit, then salty feta, hearty spinach, and crunchy almonds. There is so much flavor in this mason jar! When it's time to eat, give the mason jar a shake or pour all the ingredients into a bowl so you get a bite of everything in one forkful.

I cup quick-cooking (pearled) farro

½ cup extra-virgin olive oil

¼ cup balsamic vinegar

2 cups shredded green cabbage

2 cups chopped fresh seasonal fruit (like strawberries)

½ cup feta cheese or vegan feta

4 cups packed spinach leaves

¼ cup chopped roasted almonds

Cook the farro according to package directions, usually about 10 minutes.

In one small mason jar, combine 2 tablespoons of olive oil, 1 tablespoon of vinegar, ½ cup of cooked farro, ½ cup of cabbage, ½ cup of fruit, 2 tablespoons of feta cheese, 1 cup of spinach, and 1 tablespoon of almonds. Repeat this process with three more jars.

Seal the jars and either eat immediately or store in the fridge for up to 5 days.

PER SERVING: Calories: 470, Fat: 28g, Sat Fat: 5g, Sodium: 250mg, Carbohydrates: 47g, Dietary Fiber: 9g, Added Sugar: 0g, Protein: 11g, Vitamin D: 0mcg, Calcium: 187mg, Iron: 3mg, Potassium: 605mg

Fun Facts

Recent research suggests that marathon runners who consumed adequate amounts of unsaturated fat, iron, potassium, and magnesium performed better during their races. Plus, magnesium is involved in energy metabolism, muscle contraction, oxygen uptake, electrolyte balance, and hydration.

GRILLED STRAWBERRY AND GOAT CHEESE SANDWICH

MAKES 4 SERVINGS • **PREP TIME: 5 MINUTES / COOK TIME: 10 MINUTES**

Is there anything better than grilled crusty bread with a creamy and delicious filling? This untraditional grilled cheese has a combination of goat cheese, strawberries, basil, and balsamic vinegar for a sweet and savory sandwich. Customize the sandwich to your liking—sub in any type of soft, spreadable vegan cheese or your favorite type of bread.

2 cups sliced strawberries

2 teaspoons chopped fresh basil

2 teaspoons balsamic vinegar

8 pieces ciabatta bread

½ cup goat cheese or vegan goat cheese

2 tablespoons extra-virgin olive oil

In a small bowl, stir together the strawberries, basil, and vinegar.

Lay out one piece of bread and top with 1 tablespoon of goat cheese and a quarter of the strawberry mixture. Top with another 1 tablespoon of goat cheese and put a second piece of ciabatta bread on top. Repeat this process for three more sandwiches.

Warm the olive oil in a large frying pan over medium heat. Place the sandwiches in the pan and top with something heavy (like a pot lid) to press them down. Cook for 3 minutes, flip, then cook for 3 minutes more, until golden brown on both sides.

Serve warm.

PER SERVING: Calories: 360, Fat: 14g, Sat Fat: 4.5g, Sodium: 420mg, Carbohydrates: 50g, Dietary Fiber: 3g, Added Sugar: 2g, Protein: 10g, Vitamin D: 0mcg, Calcium: 135mg, Iron: 3mg, Potassium: 155mg

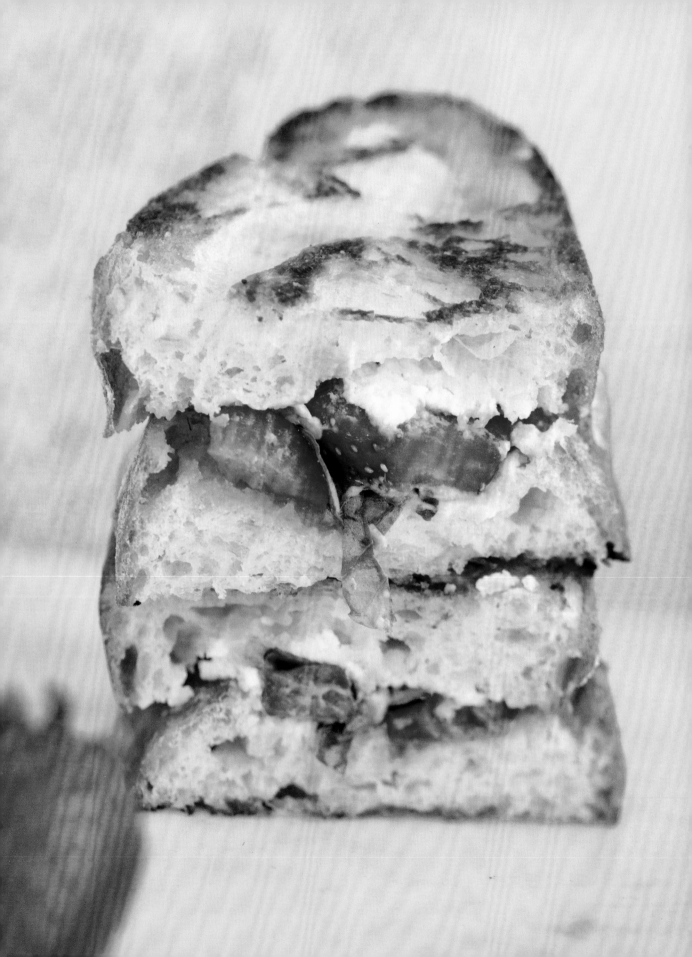

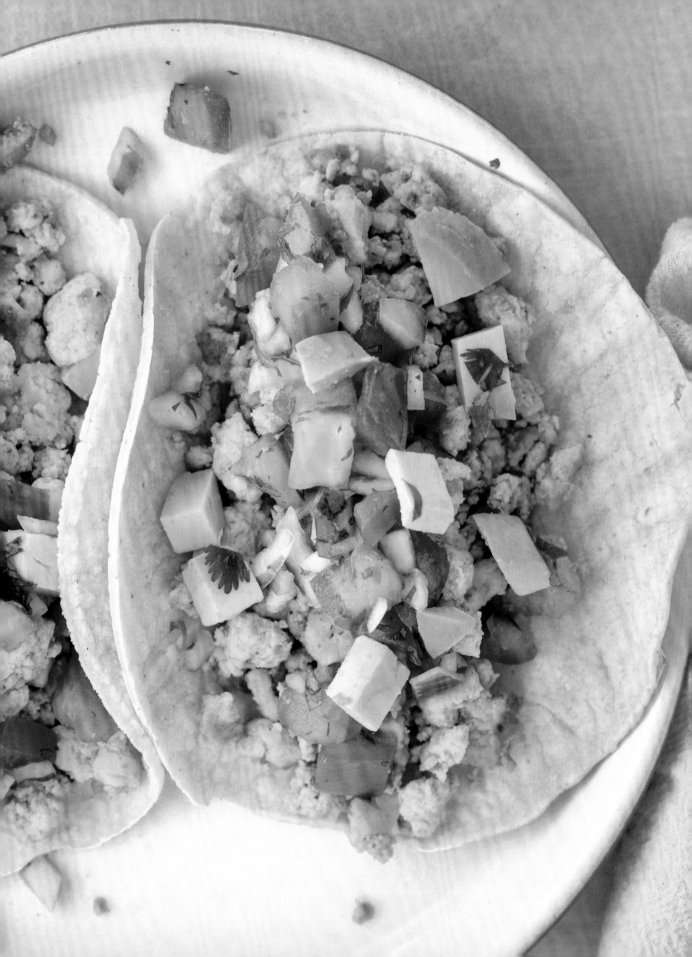

CRUMBLED TOFU RANCHEROS

MAKES 4 SERVINGS • PREP TIME: 10 MINUTES / COOK TIME: 10 MINUTES

Tofu rancheros is a completely plant-based version of the traditional eggy brunch dish. Made with crumbled tofu that has been cooked in a variety of spices, and a homemade pico de gallo, these breakfast tacos will fill you up any time of the day. Might I suggest making a quick batch of 5-Ingredient Guacamole (page 101) to serve on top?

16 ounces firm tofu, crumbled

2 teaspoons ground turmeric

1 teaspoon chili powder

½ teaspoon garlic powder

½ teaspoon salt, plus salt as needed

2 tablespoons vegetable oil

1 cup chopped tomato

½ cup chopped red onion

2 tablespoons fresh lime juice

2 tablespoons chopped fresh cilantro

8 corn tortillas, small (3 to 4 inches)

1 avocado, pitted, peeled, and chopped (optional)

Preheat the oven to 350°F.

In a large bowl, combine the tofu, turmeric, chili powder, garlic powder, and ½ teaspoon of salt. Stir until well combined.

Warm the vegetable oil a large frying pan over medium heat. Add the tofu mixture and cook, stirring for 5 minutes, until golden brown. Remove from the heat.

Meanwhile, in a small bowl, mix together the tomato, onion, lime juice, and cilantro. Season to taste with salt.

When ready to serve, place the tortillas on a baking sheet and place in the oven for 2 to 3 minutes, until warm. Remove them from the oven and top with the tofu, pico de gallo, and avocado, if using. Serve warm. Store the tofu and pico de gallo in separate sealed containers in the fridge for up to 5 days. Assemble right before eating.

PER SERVING: Calories: 360, Fat: 19g, Sat Fat: 2g, Sodium: 500mg, Carbohydrates: 36g, Dietary Fiber: 5g, Added Sugar: 0g, Protein: 16g, Vitamin D: 0mcg, Calcium: 211mg, Iron: 3mg, Potassium: 639mg

Fun Facts

You can freeze tofu to reduce the water content and increase the crispiness when cooking. Slice the tofu as per the recipe instructions, then place it in a freezer-safe bag. When ready to cook, defrost the tofu in the fridge or under warm running water.

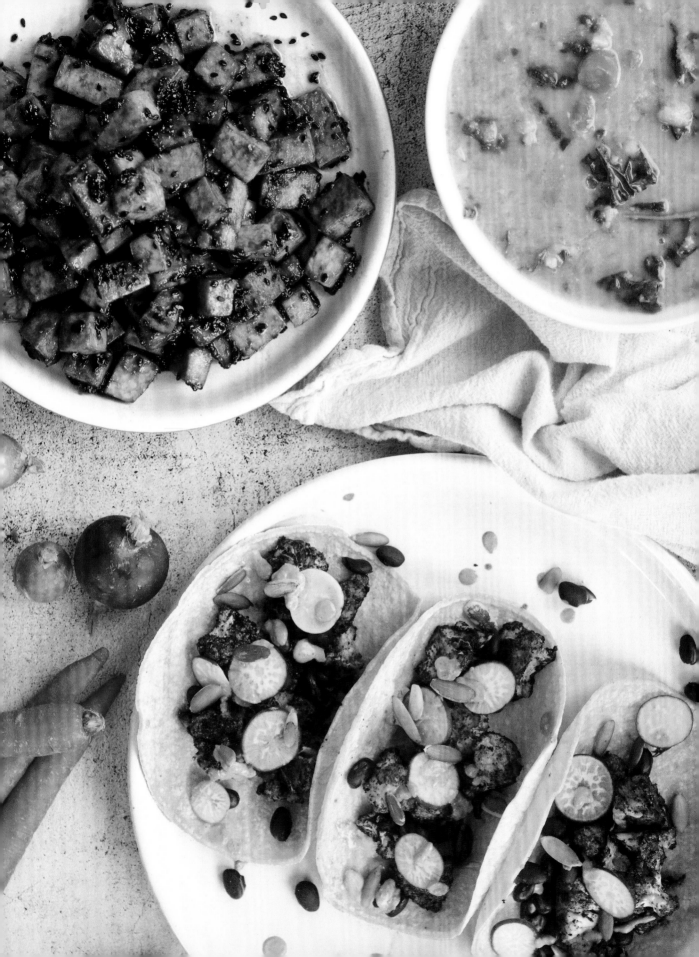

CHAPTER 5

HEARTY DINNERS

After a tough day of training, every athlete needs a hearty dinner that fills them up without weighing them down. And no surprise here—you can absolutely make a well-balanced, delicious, plant-based dinner with a mixture of all three macronutrients, vitamins, minerals, and antioxidants. These filling meatless mains will not only satisfy your taste buds but also help you refuel and recover for tomorrow's training. If you're looking to take taco night up a notch, check out the Cauliflower Tacos with Chipotle Crema (page 86). The Wild Rice and Mushroom Umami Burgers with Roasted Red Pepper Aioli (page 90) are a flavor bomb in your mouth!

GREENS AND BEANS SOUP

MAKES 4 SERVINGS • PREP TIME: 10 MINUTES / COOK TIME: 45 MINUTES

There's nothing easier than making a big pot of soup—it's the ultimate one-pot meal! This greens and beans soup combines hearty kale with protein-rich white beans, plus other veggies and herbs. White beans are a stand-out ingredient due to their nutrition profile. Not only are they a good source of plant-based protein and fiber, they are also an excellent source of iron and folate, two nutrients necessary for blood and brain health.

- 2 tablespoons extra-virgin olive oil
- 2 stalks celery, chopped (½ cup)
- 2 carrots, chopped (¾ cup)
- ¼ white onion, diced (¼ cup)
- 4 cloves garlic, minced
- I cup chopped artichoke hearts
- I teaspoon dried rosemary
- ¾ teaspoon salt
- ¼ teaspoon dried thyme
- 2 cans (15.5 oz) cannellini beans, drained and rinsed
- 4 cups low-sodium vegetable broth
- I cup water
- 2 tablespoons fresh lemon juice
- 2 cups packed chopped stemmed kale
- Salt and freshly ground black pepper

Warm the olive oil in a large stockpot over medium heat. Add the celery, carrots, onion, garlic, and artichoke hearts and cook for 3 to 4 minutes, until translucent. Add the rosemary, salt, and thyme and stir. Cook for 5 minutes.

Add the beans, broth, water, and lemon juice and bring to a boil. Reduce the heat to low, cover, and simmer for 20 minutes, until the vegetables are soft.

Using an immersion blender, blend the soup until it has reached a very chunky consistency; you should still be able to see full beans and vegetables. If you don't have an immersion blender, transfer half of the soup to a blender and blend, then put it back in the stockpot with the remaining soup.

Add the kale to the pot, increase the heat to high, and bring to a boil. Reduce the heat to low, cover, and simmer for another 10 minutes, until the kale is wilted. Season to taste with salt and black pepper.

Serve immediately or store in a sealed container in the fridge for up to 7 days or in the freezer for up to 3 months. Heat before serving.

PER SERVING: Calories: 290, Fat: 7g, Sat Fat: Ig, Sodium: 790mg, Carbohydrates: 44g, Dietary Fiber: IIg, Added Sugar: 0g, Protein: 13g, Vitamin D: 0mcg, Calcium: 157mg, Iron: 5mg, Potassium: 812mg

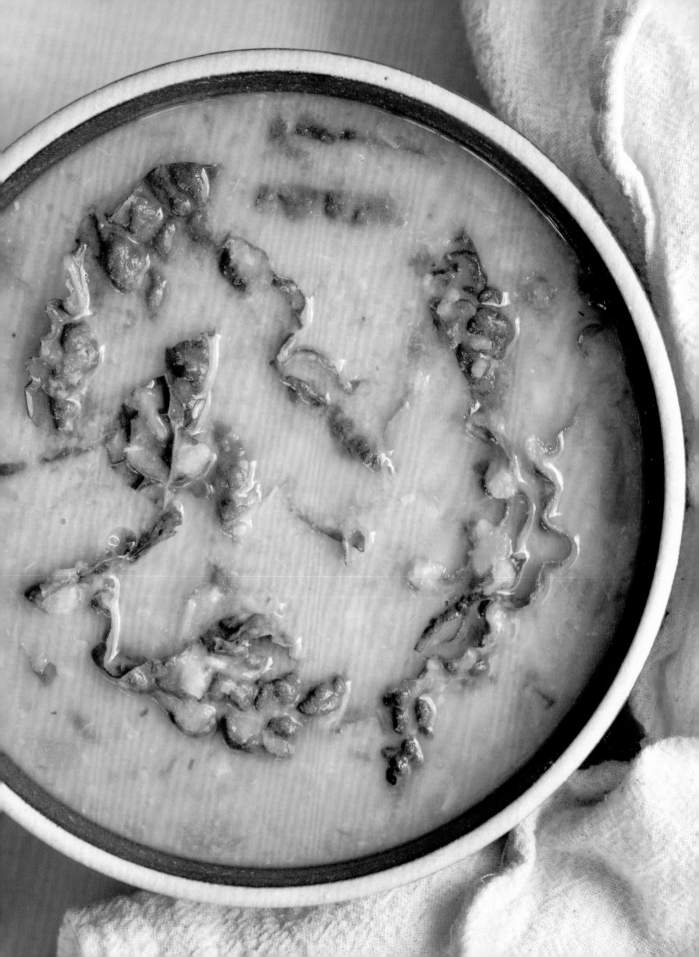

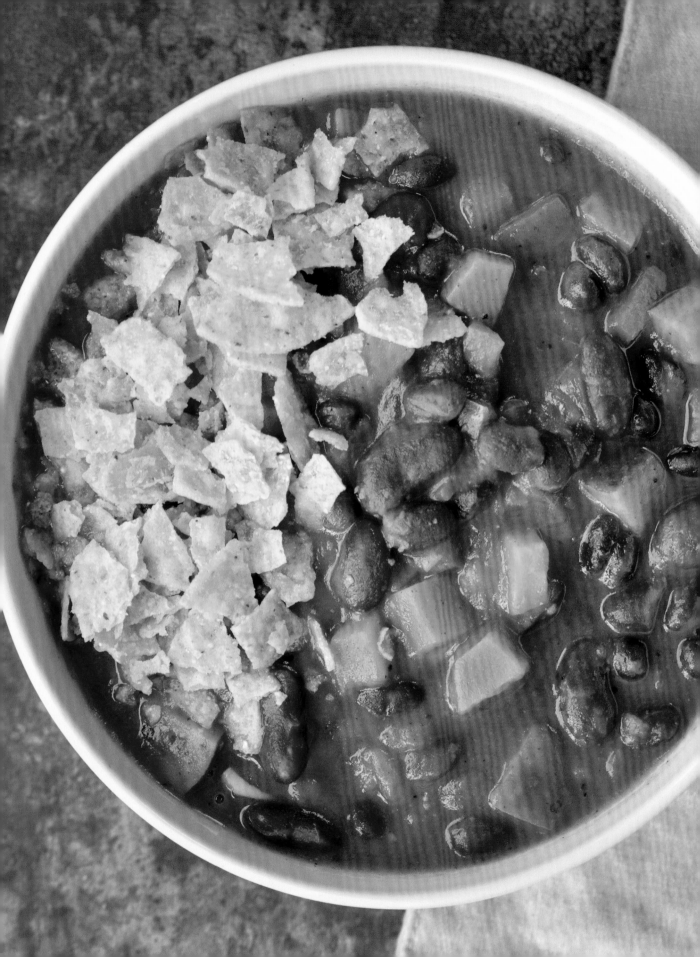

PUMPKIN CHILI

MAKES 4 SERVINGS   •   PREP TIME: 10 MINUTES / COOK TIME: 40 MINUTES

Take chili up a notch with the warm fall flavors of cinnamon and pumpkin. A bowl of this chili has everything you love about a comforting bowl of stew—veggies, beans, and rich flavors—and it's a one-pot meal that comes together in about 30 minutes. Top it with your favorite chili toppings, such as tortilla chips, sliced jalapeños, sliced green onions, or cheese.

1 tablespoon vegetable oil

1 yellow onion, diced (1 cup)

1 bell pepper, any color, chopped (1 cup)

1 sweet potato, chopped (2 cups)

3 cloves garlic, minced

2 teaspoons chili powder

1 teaspoon ground cumin

½ teaspoon salt

½ teaspoon ground cinnamon

2 cups low-sodium vegetable broth

1 cup canned crushed tomatoes

1 can (15.5 oz) 100% pumpkin puree

1 can (15.5 oz) kidney beans, drained and rinsed

1 can (15.5 oz) black beans, drained and rinsed

Warm the vegetable oil in a large stockpot over medium-high heat. Add the onion, bell pepper, sweet potato, and garlic. Cook for 3 to 5 minutes, until the onion is translucent.

Add the chili powder, cumin, salt, and cinnamon and cook for 2 to 3 minutes. Add the broth, tomatoes, pumpkin, kidney beans, and black beans and stir. Bring the mixture to a boil. Cover, reduce the heat to low, and simmer for 20 to 25 minutes, until the potatoes are fork-tender.

Serve immediately or store in a sealed container in the fridge for up to 7 days or in the freezer for up to 3 months. Heat before serving.

PER SERVING: Calories: 380, Fat: 2.5g, Sat Fat: 0g, Sodium: 490mg, Carbohydrates: 73g, Dietary Fiber: 19g, Added Sugar: 0g, Protein: 19g, Vitamin D: 0mcg, Calcium: 205mg, Iron: 6mg, Potassium: 1,118mg

Fun Facts

Your intestines absorb fat-soluble vitamins (vitamins A, D, E, and K) at a much greater rate when eaten with a healthy fat source. Try combining a sweet potato (vitamin A) with avocado (vitamin E) for max absorption.

CORN FRITTERS WITH APPLE YOGURT SAUCE

MAKES 4 SERVINGS • PREP TIME: 5 MINUTES / COOK TIME: 10 MINUTES

Fritters are traditionally made with butter and eggs and fried in tons of oil, making them an unhealthy treat. This version of corn fritters is not only vegan but also cooked in a pan with only a touch of oil—you can have the delicious chewy and sweet corn cake without all the extra grease! These yummy fritters are served with a yogurt sauce for an extra flavor boost and protein kick. Eat them with a fork and knife or pick them up with your hands and take a big bite.

FOR THE FRITTERS

2 cups unsalted corn kernels

1 large egg (see tip)

¾ cup plant-based milk

½ cup all-purpose flour

¼ cup cornmeal

2 teaspoons chopped fresh chives

½ teaspoon baking powder

½ teaspoon garlic powder

½ teaspoon salt

Freshly ground black pepper

2 tablespoons vegetable oil

FOR THE YOGURT SAUCE

¼ cup plain nonfat Greek yogurt or nondairy yogurt

½ cup shredded red apple

To make the fritters, in a large bowl, combine the corn, egg, milk, flour, cornmeal, chives, baking powder, garlic powder, and salt. Season to taste with black pepper. Whisk until well combined.

Heat the vegetable oil in a large frying pan over medium-high heat. Pour ¼ cup of batter into the pan for each pancake. Cook on one side for 3 to 4 minutes, or until golden brown. Use a spatula to flip and cook on the other side for 3 to 4 minutes longer, or until golden brown. Transfer to a paper towel–lined plate to drain.

To make the yogurt sauce, combine the yogurt and apple in a small bowl and mix well.

Serve immediately or store the fritters and yogurt sauce in separate sealed containers in the fridge for up to 3 days. Before eating, reheat with a drop of vegetable oil in a frying pan over medium-low heat for 5 minutes.

PER SERVING (2 FRITTERS PLUS 1 TABLESPOON OF SAUCE): Calories: 270, Fat: 10g, Sat Fat: 1.5g, Sodium: 360mg, Carbohydrates: 39g, Dietary Fiber: 3g, Added Sugar: 0g, Protein: 8g, Vitamin D: 1mcg, Calcium: 156mg, Iron: 1mg, Potassium: 353mg

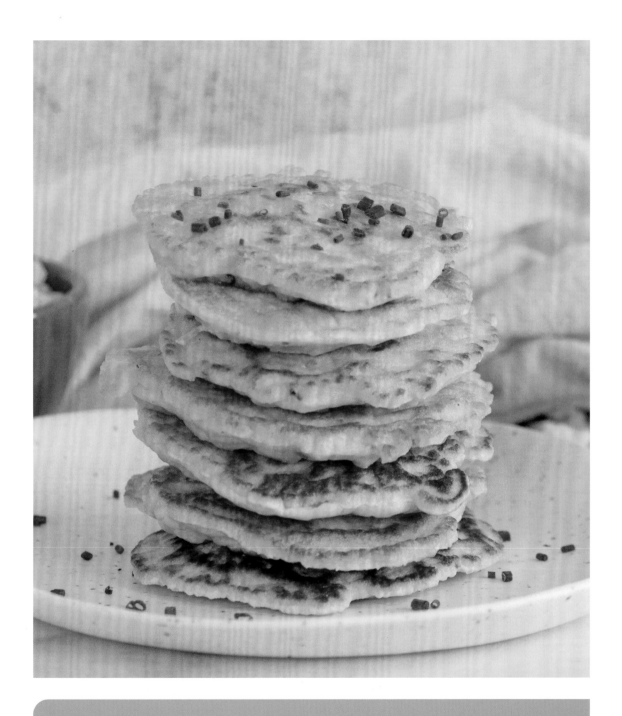

Vegan Tip: To replace the egg with a chia egg, combine 1 tablespoon of chia seeds and 3 tablespoons of water in a small bowl. Let the mixture sit for 5 minutes until a gel forms.

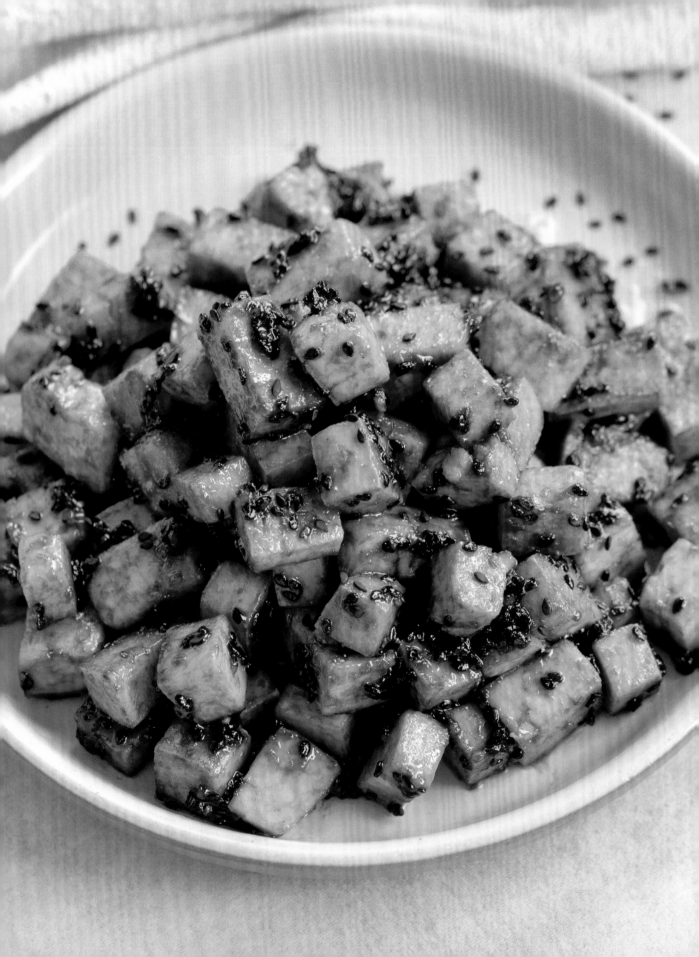

SWEET AND STICKY TOFU

MAKES 4 SERVINGS • PREP TIME: 5 MINUTES / COOK TIME: 15 MINUTES

I'll be the first to admit that tofu can be bland. But this recipe takes tofu up a notch with a sweet and tangy marinade. The best part is that you don't have to marinate it ahead of time—the sauce adds a sticky honey flavor in just minutes at the end of the cooking process. My husband ate a whole block of tofu when I made this recipe!

4 cloves garlic, minced

¼ cup low-sodium soy sauce

¼ cup light or dark brown sugar, packed

2 tablespoons sesame oil

1 teaspoon cornstarch

1 tablespoon sesame seeds

2 tablespoons vegetable oil

2 pounds tofu, cut into 1-inch cubes

In a small bowl, combine the garlic, soy sauce, brown sugar, sesame oil, cornstarch, and sesame seeds. Whisk until well combined and set the sauce aside.

Warm the vegetable oil in a large frying pan over medium heat. Add the tofu and cook for 5 minutes, until lightly golden brown. Use a spatula to flip and cook for 5 minutes longer, until the other side is golden brown.

Pour the soy sauce mixture into the pan and stir with the spatula until the tofu is well coated. Cook for 2 to 3 minutes, until the soy sauce mixture starts to caramelize, then remove the tofu from the pan.

Serve immediately or store in a sealed container in the fridge for up to 3 days.

PER SERVING: Calories: 330, Fat: 23g, Sat Fat: 3g, Sodium: 710mg, Carbohydrates: 18g, Dietary Fiber: 0g, Added Sugar: 12g, Protein: 18g, Vitamin D: 0mcg, Calcium: 270mg, Iron: 3mg, Potassium: 309mg

Fun Facts

Are you hungry all the time? If so, there's a good chance that you aren't fueling properly for or recovering from a workout. Putting the right fuel in your system not only gives you energy but also helps control the hunger that creeps up on endurance athletes.

CAULIFLOWER TACOS WITH CHIPOTLE CREMA

MAKES 12 TACOS • **PREP TIME: 10 MINUTES / COOK TIME: 35 MINUTES**

We have a standard Taco Tuesday night in my household, and my husband always requests this recipe. These cauliflower tacos are a crowd-pleaser, and they are really simple to make. The chipotle crema is made with silken tofu, rather than sour cream, for a protein punch (you can also use a 5.3-ounce container of Greek yogurt, if you prefer). After a long day of training, do yourself a favor and whip up this simple dinner, which will satisfy your hunger and taste buds.

2 heads cauliflower, cut into florets

¼ cup plus 2 tablespoons vegetable oil

2 teaspoons chili powder

I teaspoon ground cumin

½ teaspoon plus ⅛ teaspoon salt, divided

6 ounces silken tofu

2 tablespoons fresh lime juice

I clove garlic, minced

I chipotle chile

12 corn tortillas, small (3 to 4 inches)

2 cups drained and rinsed black beans

2 tablespoons pumpkin seeds (optional)

Sliced radishes or green cabbage (optional)

Preheat the oven to 375°F.

In a large bowl, combine the cauliflower, vegetable oil, chili powder, cumin, and ½ teaspoon of salt. Stir until the cauliflower is coated in the spice mixture.

Spread the cauliflower on a baking sheet and bake for 30 minutes, or until golden brown. Leave the oven on after you take out the cauliflower.

Meanwhile, make the chipotle crema. In a food processor, combine the tofu, lime juice, garlic, chipotle, and remaining ⅛ teaspoon of salt. Process until smooth.

Place the tortillas in the oven for 1 to 2 minutes, until warm.

Assemble the tacos. Add the cauliflower mixture to the tortillas, then top with the beans, pumpkin seeds, if using, and radishes, if using. Serve with a drizzle of crema.

PER SERVING (3 TACOS): Calories: 460, Fat: 25g, Sat Fat: 3.5g, Sodium: 540mg, Carbohydrates: 55g, Dietary Fiber: 7g, Added Sugar: 0g, Protein: 13g, Vitamin D: 0mcg, Calcium: 179mg, Iron: 3mg, Potassium: 1,169mg

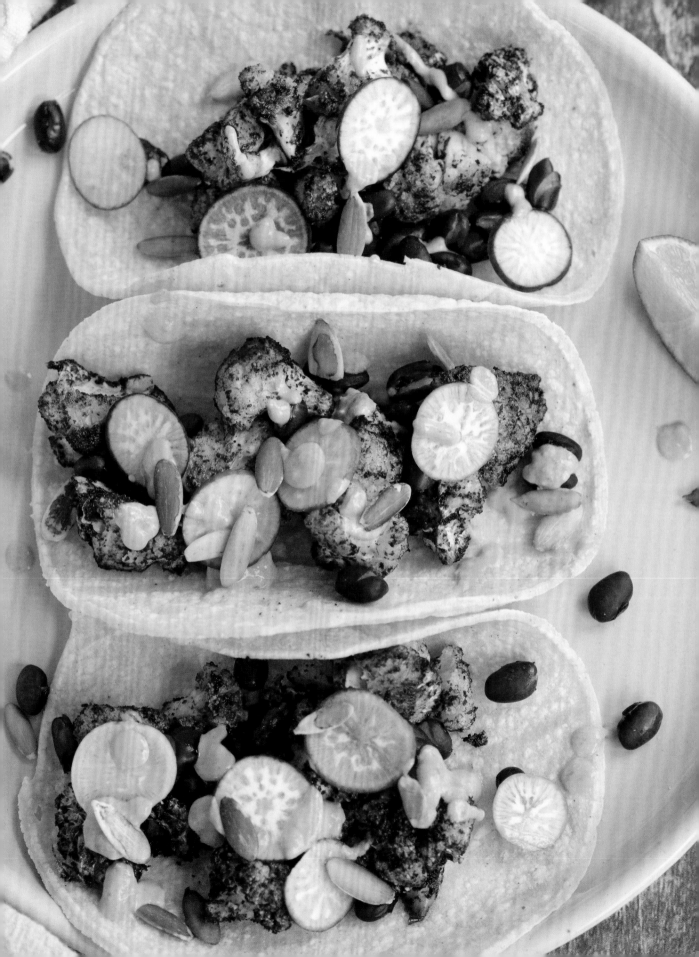

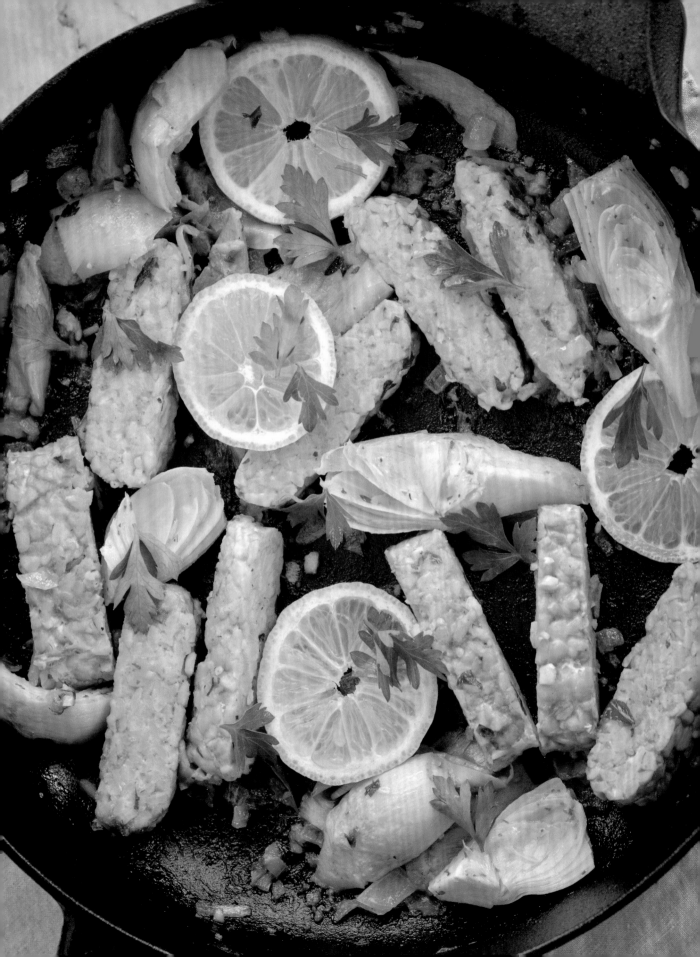

TEMPEH WITH LEMON AND ARTICHOKES

MAKES 4 SERVINGS • **PREP TIME: 5 MINUTES / COOK TIME: 15 MINUTES**

My mom used to make a delicious chicken with artichokes that was served in a tangy white wine sauce. When I went plant-based, it was one of the dishes I missed the most. But luckily for me, tempeh has a "meaty" flavor that makes it the perfect protein stand-in for this dish. If you're unfamiliar with tempeh, it's a fermented soybean product that usually comes in a block form. It's loaded with good-for-your-gut probiotics, and it usually only requires a little bit of marinade for simple cooking. Case in point, this tasty tempeh dish is cooked in one pan with artichokes, lemon juice, and vegetable broth.

2 tablespoons extra-virgin olive oil

1 cup chopped white onion

4 cloves garlic, minced

2 cups marinated artichokes

¼ cup fresh lemon juice

3 cups low-sodium vegetable broth

16 ounces tempeh, cut into 2-inch slices

Salt and freshly ground black pepper

2 tablespoons chopped fresh flat-leaf parsley

In a cast iron or nonstick frying pan over medium-high heat, combine the olive oil, onion, and garlic. Cook for 2 to 3 minutes, until the onion is translucent.

Add the artichokes, lemon juice, broth, and tempeh. Cook for 5 minutes, then flip the tempeh and cook for 5 minutes longer, until some of the liquid evaporates. Season to taste with salt and black pepper.

Top with the parsley and serve immediately. Store leftovers in a sealed container in the fridge for up to 3 days.

PER SERVING: Calories: 380, Fat: 26g, Sat Fat: 4.5g, Sodium: 610mg, Carbohydrates: 18g, Dietary Fiber: 2g, Added Sugar: 0g, Protein: 26g, Vitamin D: 0mcg, Calcium: 163mg, Iron: 3mg, Potassium: 568mg

Fun Facts

To reduce the bitterness of tempeh, cover it with water in a small pot. Bring it to a boil, then reduce the heat to low and simmer for 10 minutes. Proceed to cook according to the recipe instructions.

WILD RICE AND MUSHROOM UMAMI BURGERS WITH ROASTED RED PEPPER AIOLI

MAKES 4 SERVINGS • PREP TIME: 10 MINUTES, PLUS 1 HOUR TO CHILL / COOK TIME: 15 MINUTES

I'm not sure what I like most about this recipe—the umami flavor of the burgers or the tangy taste of the red pepper aioli. The combination of the two really can't be beat! These burgers combine savory ingredients, like wild rice, mushroom, walnuts, and soy sauce with a vibrant vegetable sauce. If you prefer to use an egg in place of the flax meal mixture, go right ahead!

FOR THE PATTIES

2 tablespoons flax meal

6 tablespoons warm water

2 tablespoons vegetable oil, divided

½ cup diced white onion

2 cloves garlic, minced

1 cup diced white mushrooms

¼ cup raw unsalted walnuts, finely chopped

2 tablespoons low-sodium soy sauce

½ teaspoon ground cumin

1½ cups cooked wild rice

½ cup panko bread crumbs

FOR THE ROASTED RED PEPPER AIOLI

½ cup mayonnaise or vegan mayonnaise

¼ cup roasted red bell peppers

1 clove garlic

⅛ teaspoon salt

To make the patties, in a small bowl, make a flax egg by combining the flax meal and water. Let sit for at least 5 minutes, until the mixture thickens slightly.

Warm 1 tablespoon of vegetable oil in a large frying pan over medium heat. Add the onion and garlic and cook for 2 to 3 minutes, until the onion is translucent. Add the mushrooms, walnuts, soy sauce, and cumin and cook for 3 to 4 minutes, until the soy sauce reduces. Remove from the heat.

In a large bowl, combine the flax egg with the vegetable mixture. Add the wild rice and bread crumbs. Mix until well combined.

Line a baking sheet with parchment paper. Form four equal patties from the mixture and place them on the prepared baking sheet. Refrigerate for at least 1 hour to set.

While the burgers are setting, make the aioli. In a food processor, combine the mayonnaise, roasted red bell peppers, garlic, and salt and process until smooth.

Heat the remaining 1 tablespoon of vegetable oil in the same large frying pan over medium-high heat. Place the burgers in the pan and cook for 4 minutes on each side, until they are golden brown.

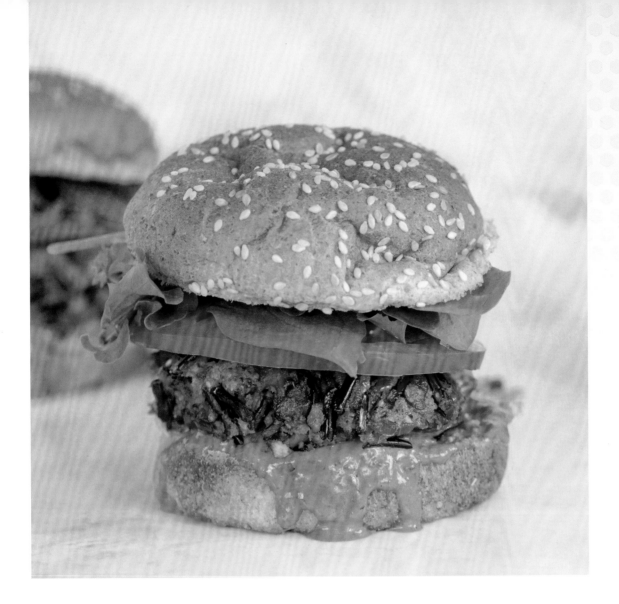

4 hamburger buns, for serving

Lettuce, for serving

Sliced tomato, for serving

To assemble, spread the aioli sauce on the bottom buns, place the patties on the buns, then top with lettuce and tomato. Serve right away or store in a sealed container in the fridge for up to 5 days or in the freezer for up to 1 month.

PER SERVING: Calories: 410, Fat: 33g, Sat Fat: 4.5g, Sodium: 690mg, Carbohydrates: 24g, Dietary Fiber: 3g, Added Sugar: 0g, Protein: 7g, Vitamin D: 0mcg, Calcium: 27mg, Iron: 1mg, Potassium: 200mg

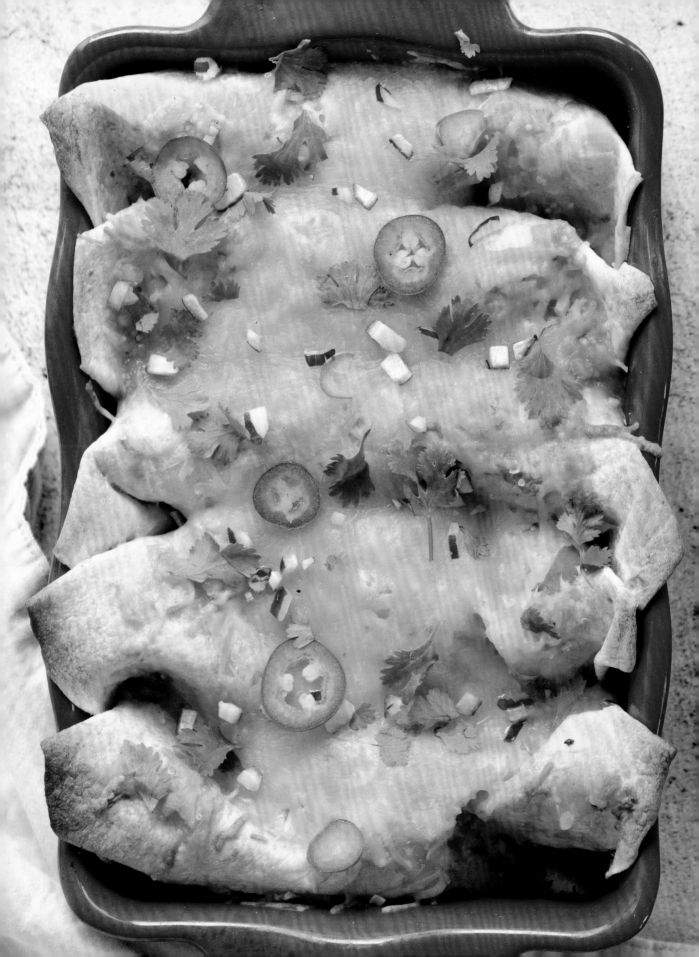

SWEET POTATO AND BLACK BEAN ENCHILADAS

MAKES 4 SERVINGS • PREP TIME: 10 MINUTES / COOK TIME: 1 HOUR

Enchiladas may seem like a complicated dish but making them at home is easier than you think. This version combines sweet potatoes, black beans, and cauliflower, rolled up in a tortilla and coated with a green salsa and cheese. Feel free to use vegan cheese.

- I sweet potato, cut into large chunks
- I cup chopped cauliflower (about ½ small head)
- ⅓ cup diced red onion, plus more for serving
- I tablespoon diced jalapeño, plus slices for serving
- 2 cloves garlic, minced
- 2 tablespoons vegetable oil
- I teaspoon chili powder
- ¼ teaspoon ground cumin
- ¼ teaspoon salt
- I can (15.5 oz) black beans, drained and rinsed
- 2 tablespoons fresh lime juice
- 6 (8- to 10-inch) soft flour tortillas
- ½ cup salsa verde
- ½ cup shredded Cheddar cheese, Mexican cheese blend, or vegan cheddar
- Diced red onion, for serving
- Sliced jalapeño, for serving
- Chopped fresh cilantro, for serving

Preheat the oven to 375°F. Line a baking sheet with parchment paper.

Bring a large pot of water to a boil over high heat. Add the sweet potato and cook for 20 minutes, until fork-tender. Drain the water and set the sweet potato aside. Remove the skins from the sweet potatoes when cool enough to handle and place the flesh in a large bowl. Mash the flesh with a fork.

Meanwhile, in another large bowl, combine the cauliflower, onion, jalapeño, garlic, vegetable oil, chili powder, cumin, and salt. Stir until well combined. Spread the cauliflower mixture on the prepared baking sheet and bake for 20 minutes, until golden around the edges.

Transfer the roasted cauliflower back to the large bowl. Add the mashed sweet potato, black beans, and lime juice and stir well.

Lay each tortilla flat and fill the middle of each tortilla with the vegetable mixture before rolling them up.

Place half of the salsa in the bottom of a 9 × 13-inch casserole dish. Place each filled tortilla in the casserole dish, with the rolled part facing down. Add the remaining half of the salsa and sprinkle cheese on top. Bake for 20 minutes, until the cheese is fully melted.

Remove the enchiladas from the oven and garnish.

PER SERVING: Calories: 470, Fat: 17g, Sat Fat: 5g, Sodium: 970mg, Carbohydrates: 61g, Dietary Fiber: 9g, Added Sugar: 1g, Protein: 14g, Vitamin D: 0mcg, Calcium: 266mg, Iron: 3mg, Potassium: 737mg

SPAGHETTI SQUASH WITH LENTIL "MEATBALLS"

MAKES 4 SERVINGS • **PREP TIME: 10 MINUTES / COOK TIME: 60 MINUTES**

I grew up in an Italian American family, so meatballs were a staple in my house. We ate them on an almost weekly basis, and they always graced our holiday table. When I switched to a plant-based diet, I wanted to create a plant-based meatball that tastes just as good as the ones my family made. These lentil meatballs have a "meaty" flavor and are loaded with veggies, cheese (or nutritional yeast), and bread crumbs. They're vegan, but if you'd like, you can replace the flax eggs with two eggs. I serve these "meatballs" over roasted spaghetti squash for a lighter weeknight dinner.

- 1 spaghetti squash, halved lengthwise and seeded
- 3 tablespoons extra-virgin olive oil, divided
- Salt and freshly ground black pepper
- 2 tablespoons flax meal
- 6 tablespoons warm water
- 1 large carrot, chopped (½ cup)
- ½ white onion, chopped (½ cup)
- 3 cloves garlic, minced
- 2 cups cooked lentils
- ½ cup seasoned bread crumbs
- 2 tablespoons chopped fresh basil
- 1 teaspoon dried oregano
- ½ teaspoon salt
- ¼ cup vegetarian parmesan cheese or nutritional yeast
- 1 cup healthy sauce of choice, for serving

Preheat the oven to 400°F.

Place the spaghetti squash on a baking sheet and drizzle with 1 tablespoon of olive oil. Season to taste with salt and black pepper. Bake, flipping the squash halfway through, for 30 minutes, until fork-tender. Remove from the oven and set aside. Keep the oven on.

Meanwhile, in a small bowl, make a flax egg by combining the flax meal and water. Let sit for at least 5 minutes, until the mixture thickens slightly.

Warm 1 tablespoon of olive oil in a medium frying pan over medium heat. Add the carrot, onion, and garlic. Cook for 5 minutes, until the onion is translucent.

In a large bowl, combine the flax egg, vegetable mixture, lentils, bread crumbs, basil, oregano, salt, and the parmesan. Use a large spoon to mix well.

Reduce the oven temperature to 350°F. Line a baking sheet with parchment paper.

Use your hands to form meatballs (a little larger than a golf ball) from the lentil mixture and place them on the prepared baking sheet. Drizzle the remaining 1 tablespoon of olive oil on top of the meatballs.

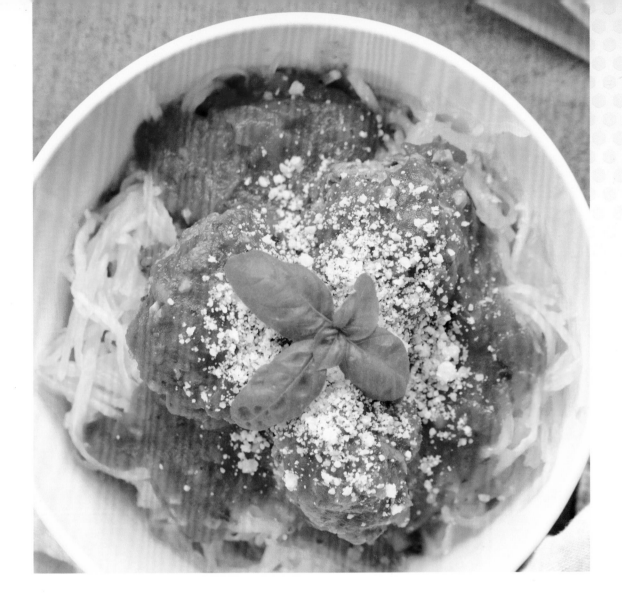

Bake, turning the meatballs halfway through, for 25 minutes, until golden and slightly crisp around edges.

Meanwhile, using a fork, scrape the flesh out of the spaghetti squash. Serve the meatballs on top of the squash with your favorite sauce, warmed for serving. Serve immediately or store the meatballs and spaghetti squash in separate sealed containers in the fridge for up to 5 days or in the freezer for up to 1 month.

PER SERVING: Calories: 450, Fat: 22g, Sat Fat: 2.5g, Sodium: 1070mg , Carbohydrates: 48g, Dietary Fiber: 13g, Added Sugar: 4g, Protein: 17g, Vitamin D: 0mcg, Calcium: 170mg, Iron: 5mg, Potassium: 1052 mg

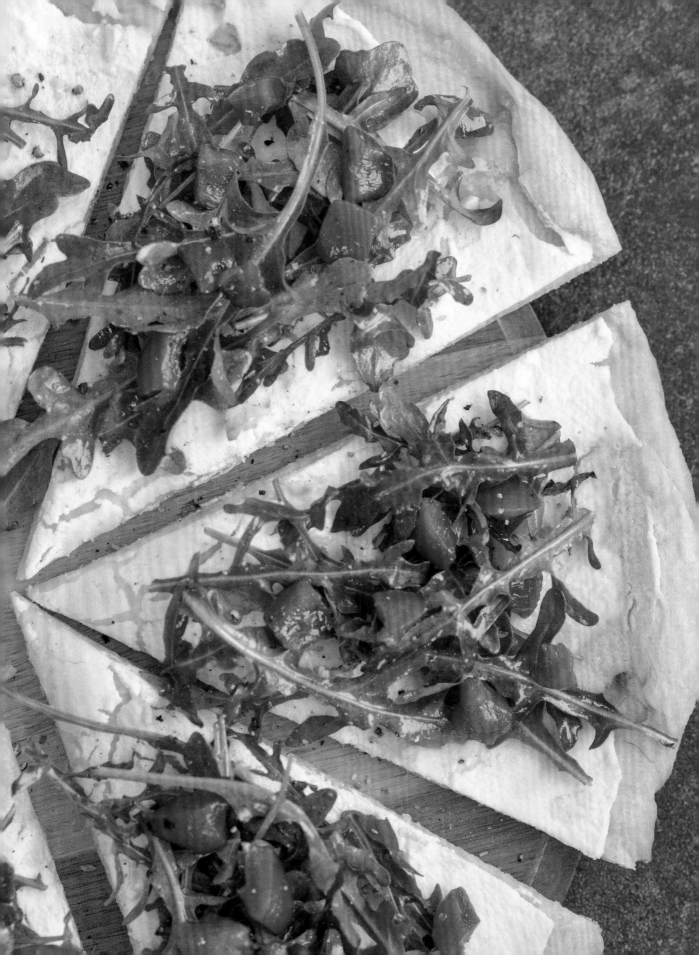

WHITE PIZZA TOPPED WITH ARUGULA SALAD

MAKES 4 SERVINGS • PREP TIME: 5 MINUTES / COOK TIME: 20 MINUTES

Making pizza at home is easier than you might think. This recipe transforms a traditional comfort food to a healthy dinner with tons of greens. My time-saving tip: Buy a store-bought dough, rather than attempt to make one from scratch. This sauceless pizza is baked with protein-packed ricotta cheese, then covered with a simple arugula salad. The bitterness of the arugula pairs nicely with the creaminess of the ricotta cheese, and it's all topped off with a hint of sweet roasted red bell peppers, olive oil, and balsamic vinegar.

- 1 tablespoon all-purpose or semolina flour
- 16 ounces store-bought pizza dough
- Cooking spray
- 1 cup part-skim ricotta cheese or vegan ricotta
- 2 cloves garlic, minced
- 3 tablespoons extra-virgin olive oil, divided
- 1 tablespoon balsamic vinegar
- ¼ teaspoon salt, plus salt as needed
- 3 cups packed arugula
- ⅓ cup chopped roasted red bell peppers
- Freshly ground black pepper

Preheat the oven to 400°F.

Spread the flour on a clean surface. Place the pizza dough on top and use your hands to evenly spread the dough to the size of a baking sheet or pizza pan.

Coat a baking sheet with cooking spray and lay the dough on top. Bake for 5 minutes, letting the dough rise. Remove the dough from the oven.

When the dough is cool enough to touch, use a spatula to spread the ricotta cheese on top. Sprinkle the garlic and 1 tablespoon of olive oil on the cheese. Bake for 10 to 12 minutes, until the pizza crust becomes golden on the bottom.

While the pizza bakes, in a large bowl, whisk together the remaining 2 tablespoons of olive oil, the vinegar, and ¼ teaspoon of salt. Add the arugula and roasted red bell peppers and toss well. Season to taste with salt and black pepper.

Place the arugula salad on top of the cooked pizza and serve immediately. Store leftover pizza, arugula, and dressing in separate sealed containers in the fridge for up to 3 days.

PER SERVING: Calories: 450, Fat: 19g, Sat Fat: 6g, Sodium: 970mg, Carbohydrates: 54g, Dietary Fiber 0g, Added Sugar: 6g, Protein: 14g, Vitamin D: 0mcg, Calcium: 197mg, Iron: 4mg, Potassium: 520mg

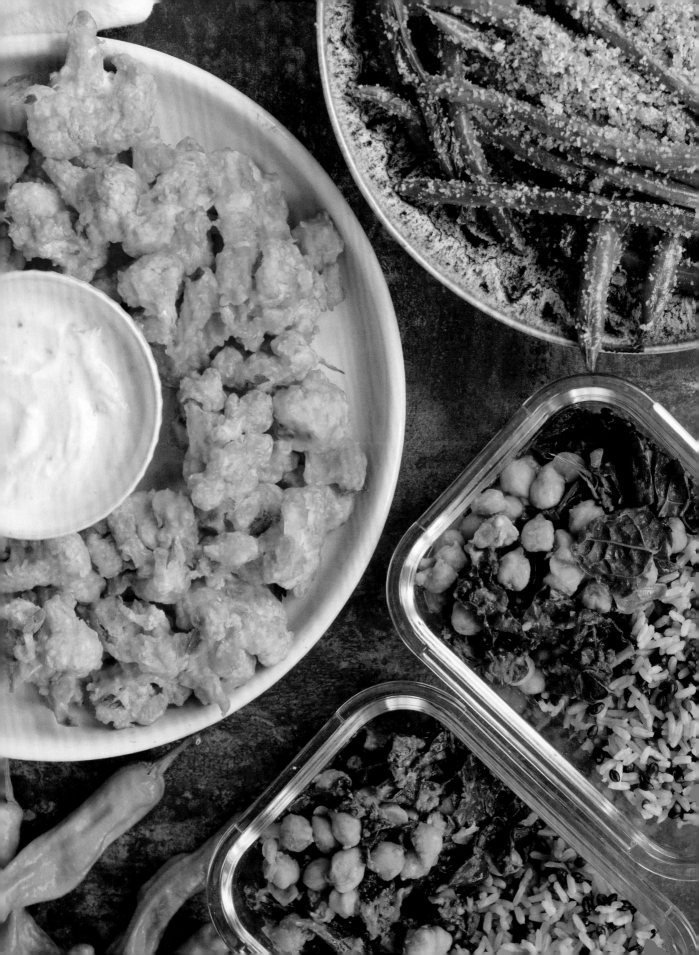

CHAPTER 6

SIDE DISHES AND DIPS

These veggie-forward side dishes amp up the nutrients of any lunch or main dish. Every single recipe in this chapter has only a few ingredients, but it showcases nature's candy in the best light. Better yet, every single side dish can be paired with other recipes. Some of my favorites? The simple Yogurt Ranch Dip (page 100) with chopped veggies is a go-to protein-packed snack that will make you ditch the bottled stuff. I make my famous 5-Ingredient Guacamole (page 101) for almost every single family gathering, and it's a huge crowd-pleaser. And the Sweet Chile Brussels Sprouts (page 109) are spicy, sticky, and sweet, making them the perfect pairing for any grain or protein.

YOGURT RANCH DIP

MAKES 4 SERVINGS • **PREP TIME: 5 MINUTES**

You won't believe how easy it is to make your own ranch dip at home. Start with yogurt, add a dash of vinegar and a pinch of herbs and seasonings, and you've got a homemade dip that is packed with protein and way healthier than a store-bought version. Put this on salads or veggie burgers, or serve with crudités or crackers. And if you don't do dairy, this tastes just as good with a plain nondairy yogurt.

¾ cup plain nonfat Greek yogurt or nondairy yogurt

1½ tablespoons apple cider vinegar

1½ teaspoons dried chives

½ teaspoon garlic powder

¼ teaspoon onion powder

¼ teaspoon salt

In a small bowl, mix together the yogurt, vinegar, chives, garlic powder, onion powder, and salt.

Serve immediately or store in a sealed container in the fridge for up to 5 days.

PER SERVING: Calories: 25, Fat: 0g, Sat Fat: 0g, Sodium: 160mg, Carbohydrates: 2g, Dietary Fiber: 0g, Added Sugar: 0g, Protein: 4g, Vitamin D: 0mcg, Calcium: 48mg, Iron: 0mg, Potassium: 73mg

Fun Facts

Both Greek yogurt and plant-based yogurt are made with live active cultures that are beneficial for gut health. A healthy gut microbiome is important for athletes because it helps supply muscles with necessary nutrients and oxygen, and it controls the transport of electrolytes through the gut lining.

5-INGREDIENT GUACAMOLE

MAKES 4 SERVINGS • PREP TIME: 5 MINUTES

Everyone needs a good guacamole recipe for entertaining guests or for just noshing on a snack filled with healthy fats. The best thing about guacamole is that it has a veggie-forward ingredient list that still tastes like an indulgent treat. Avocados are the only fruit with monounsaturated "good" fat, making them the perfect postworkout food for keeping you full. I suggest adding a dollop of this guacamole to Cauliflower Tacos with Chipotle Crema (page 86) or Sweet Potato and Black Bean Enchiladas (page 93)!

2 avocados, pitted and peeled

1 small plum tomato, diced

2 tablespoons chopped red onion

1 tablespoon fresh lime juice

½ small jalapeño, diced

¼ teaspoon salt

In a small bowl, combine the avocado, tomato, onion, lime juice, jalapeño, and salt. Using a spoon, stir all the ingredients until the avocado is mashed but still chunky.

Eat immediately or store in a sealed contained in the fridge for up to 1 day. (The guacamole will brown if left in the fridge overnight, but it's still okay to eat.)

PER SERVING: Calories: 120, Fat: 11g, Sat Fat: 1.5g, Sodium: 150mg, Carbohydrates: 8g, Dietary Fiber: 5g, Added Sugar: 0g, Protein: 2g, Vitamin D: 0mcg, Calcium: 12mg, Iron: 0mg, Potassium: 393mg

Fun Facts

A ripe avocado is darker in color and slightly soft, but not mushy. If your avocado is dark but still feels hard, leave it on the counter for a day or two to ripen. Use a ripe avocado immediately or store in the fridge for 1 to 2 days.

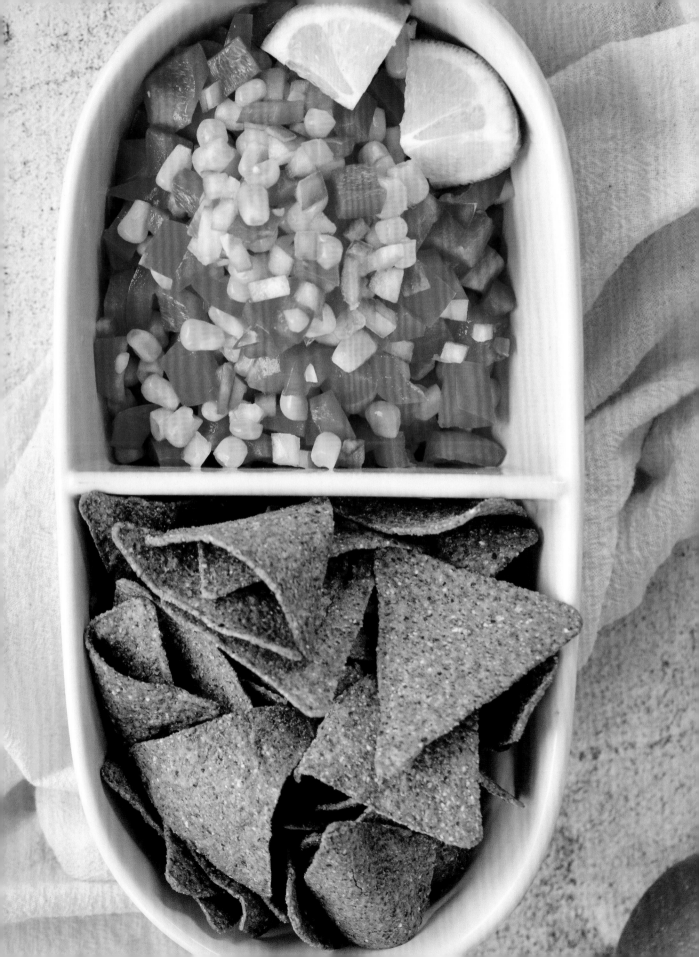

CORN AND RED PEPPER SALSA

MAKES 4 SERVINGS • **PREP TIME: 5 MINUTES**

Eating your veggies has never tasted so good! This vibrant and tasty salsa is made with just four plant-based ingredients, and it comes together in 5 minutes flat. Other than the few minutes to chop the pepper and onion, this salsa requires very little prep work and it's sure to delight your taste buds. The combination of savory onion and lime juice with sweet corn and bell pepper is a definite winner. Add a scoop of this colorful salsa to spice up the Black Bean Quesadillas (page 63).

1 red bell pepper, chopped (about 1½ cups)

1 cup unsalted corn kernels

¼ cup chopped red onion

2 tablespoons fresh lime juice

¼ teaspoon salt

In a large bowl, combine the bell pepper, corn, onion, lime juice, and salt. Mix well.

Serve immediately or store in a sealed container in the fridge for up to 5 days.

PER SERVING: Calories: 50, Fat: 0.5g, Sat Fat: 0g, Sodium: 230mg, Carbohydrates: 11g, Dietary Fiber: 2g, Added Sugar: 0g, Protein: 2g, Vitamin D: 0mcg, Calcium: 9mg, Iron: 0mg, Potassium: 196mg

Fun Facts

Corn gets a bad reputation, but it's actually packed with nutrients. It has phytochemicals, like lutein and zeaxanthin, which are beneficial for eye and brain health. It also has insoluble fiber, which aids in digestion, as well as B vitamins, iron, and potassium.

QUICK-PICKLED MIXED VEGGIES

MAKES 4 SERVINGS • **PREP TIME: 5 MINUTES, PLUS 24 HOURS TO PICKLE / COOK TIME: 10 MINUTES**

Did you know that you can easily pickle your own vegetables without any tedious canning or jarring? Better yet, you can pickle vegetables other than cucumbers! All it takes is some chopped veggies, a sweet and salty brine, and a day. And for all the heavy sweaters out there, pickled veggies replace sodium lost in sweat. So, if you work out in a hot climate, enjoy a few pieces of pickled veggies postworkout to get your electrolytes and help with hydration.

1 cup water

2 tablespoons sugar

2 cups chopped mixed vegetables, such as celery, carrots, radish, and cauliflower

1 cup apple cider vinegar

1 tablespoon salt

1 tablespoon pickling spice

In a small saucepan, bring the water and sugar to a boil over high heat. Reduce the heat to low and simmer for 10 minutes, until the sugar is dissolved.

Place the veggies in a large mason jar. Pour the water and sugar solution into the jar, and then add the vinegar, salt, and pickling spice. Put the lid on the jar and shake well.

Refrigerate for at least 24 hours before serving. Store in the fridge for up to 1 month.

PER SERVING: Calories: 60, Fat: 1g, Sat Fat: 0g, Sodium: 3,520mg, Carbohydrates: 12g, Dietary Fiber: 2g, Added Sugar: 6g, Protein: 2g, Vitamin D: 0mcg, Calcium: 47mg, Iron: 1mg, Potassium: 211mg

Fun Facts

Fermented plant-based foods, such as tempeh, miso, sauerkraut, and pickles, contribute to a healthy gut micro-biome. Having a healthy gut has been linked to increased athletic performance.

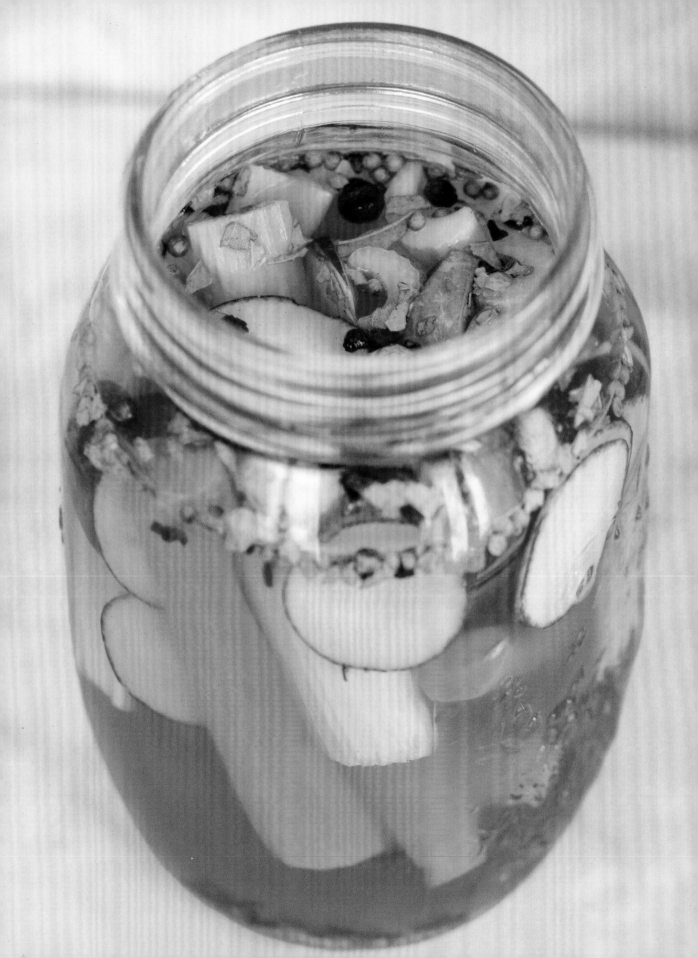

TERIYAKI MUSHROOMS

MAKES 4 SERVINGS • **PREP TIME: 5 MINUTES / COOK TIME: 10 MINUTES**

Mushrooms have a meaty texture and umami flavor, making them a staple of any plant-based diet. This side dish combines the savory flavor of mushrooms with the sweet tanginess of teriyaki sauce. This recipe uses standard white button mushrooms, but feel free to sub in your favorite variety. Add a serving of rice and cooked tofu to easily turn this side into a meal.

- 2 tablespoons neutral oil (canola, vegetable or grapeseed)
- 4 cups sliced white mushrooms
- 1 teaspoon minced fresh ginger
- 1 clove garlic, minced
- ¼ teaspoon salt
- ¼ cup teriyaki sauce

Warm the neutral oil in a large sauté pan over medium heat. Add the mushrooms, ginger, garlic, and salt. Cook for 5 minutes, until the mushrooms are golden brown.

Reduce the heat to medium-low and add the teriyaki sauce. Cook for 5 minutes longer, until most of the sauce has been absorbed into the mushrooms.

Serve immediately or store in a sealed container in the fridge for up to 5 days.

PER SERVING: Calories: 100, Fat: 7g, Sat Fat: 0.5g, Sodium: 880mg, Carbohydrates: 7g, Dietary Fiber: 1g, Added Sugar: 3g, Protein: 5g, Vitamin D: 0mcg, Calcium: 6mg, Iron: 1mg, Potassium: 44mg

Fun Facts

Vitamin D is necessary for bone health, immune system function, and inflammation prevention, yet it's difficult to get it on a plant-based diet. Mushrooms are one of the only plant-based foods with vitamin D, so many athletes turn to supplementation.

GARLICKY GREEN BEANS

MAKES 4 SERVINGS • PREP TIME: 5 MINUTES / COOK TIME: 15 MINUTES

This garlic-forward side is a filling way to eat your greens. Green beans have protein and vitamin C and are packed with fiber. Just a little bit of flavor goes a long way in making these green beans something you're going to want to eat on repeat. The flavors of this simple side pair nicely with the Sweet and Sticky Tofu (page 85). Add a grain to make it a complete meal.

2 tablespoons extra-virgin olive oil

1 pound green beans

4 cloves garlic, minced

¼ teaspoon salt

¼ cup bread crumbs

Warm the olive oil in a large sauté pan over medium-low heat. Add the green beans, spreading them evenly. Cook for 10 minutes, until the green beans are slightly charred.

Add the garlic, salt, and bread crumbs and cook for 5 minutes longer, until the bread crumbs are golden brown.

Serve immediately or store in a sealed container in the fridge for up to 5 days.

PER SERVING: Calories: 120, Fat: 7g, Sat Fat: 1g, Sodium: 190mg, Carbohydrates: 13g, Dietary Fiber: 3g, Added Sugar: 0g, Protein: 3g, Vitamin D: 0mcg, Calcium: 56mg, Iron: 2mg, Potassium: 262mg

Fun Facts

Vitamin C increases iron absorption, while phytates (present in grains and beans) and certain polyphenols in some nonanimal foods (such as cereals and legumes) interfere with the absorption of iron.

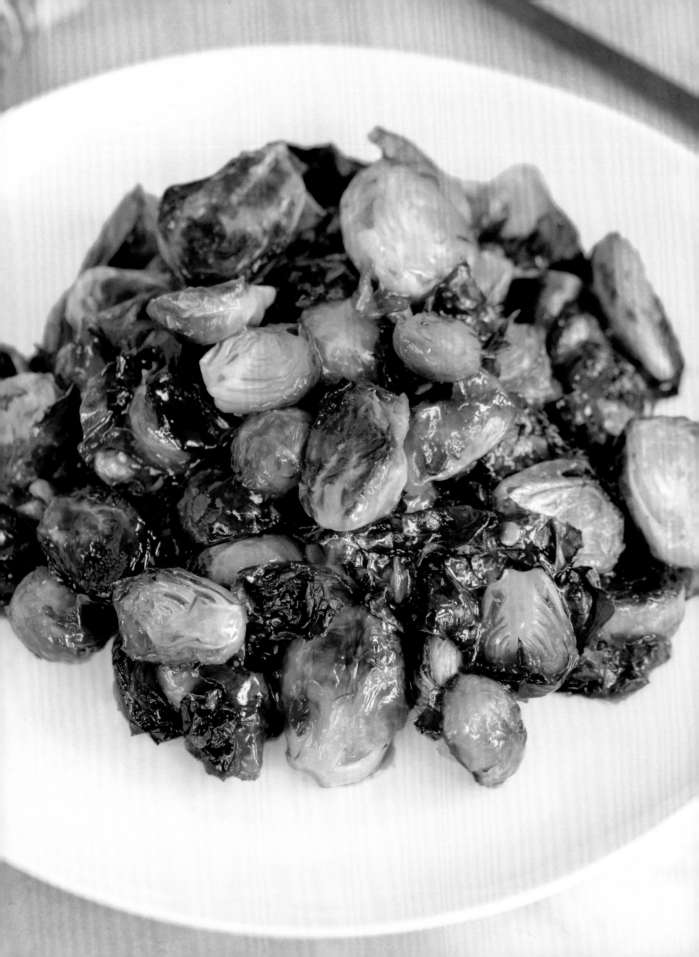

SWEET CHILE BRUSSELS SPROUTS

MAKES 4 SERVINGS • PREP TIME: 5 MINUTES / COOK TIME: 30 MINUTES

This side dish is for those who like to kick up the heat a notch. The sauce is made from a chile-garlic sauce that can be found in the international section of most supermarkets. If you aren't a huge spice fan, use ½ tablespoon of chile-garlic sauce. Brussels sprouts are full of vitamin C and fiber, so you'll also get a nice nutrient boost on top of the pop of flavor. Serve these sprouts with a simple grain to neutralize the heat.

1½ pounds brussels sprouts, stemmed and halved

2 tablespoons neutral oil (canola, vegetable, or grapeseed)

¼ teaspoon salt

½ tablespoon cornstarch

1 tablespoon plus ¼ cup water, divided

¼ cup rice vinegar

2 tablespoons sugar

1 tablespoon chile-garlic sauce

Preheat the oven to 375°F. Line a baking sheet with parchment paper.

In a large bowl, toss together the sprouts, neutral oil, and salt. Transfer the sprouts to the prepared baking sheet, spreading them evenly. Bake for 30 minutes, until crisp and brown around the edges.

Meanwhile, place the cornstarch and 1 tablespoon of water in a small bowl and stir well. Set aside.

In a large sauté pan over high heat, bring the vinegar, sugar, and remaining ¼ cup of water to a boil, stirring until the sugar dissolves, about 3 minutes. Add the cornstarch mixture, reduce the heat to low, and simmer until the sauce thickens, about 2 minutes.

Remove the pan from the heat. Add the cooked sprouts, tossing to coat in the sauce. Serve immediately or store in a sealed container in the fridge for up to 3 days.

PER SERVING: Calories: 170, Fat: 8g, Sat Fat: 0.5g, Sodium: 260mg, Carbohydrates: 23g, Dietary Fiber: 6g, Added Sugar: 6g, Protein: 6g, Vitamin D: 0mcg, Calcium: 72mg, Iron: 2mg, Potassium: 662mg

SPICED CHICKPEAS AND GREENS

MAKES 4 SERVINGS • **PREP TIME: 5 MINUTES / COOK TIME: 15 MINUTES**

Two simple ingredients—chickpeas and kale—come together to create a side that is chock-full of nutrients, such as protein, fiber, and vitamin C. This hearty side has big smoky flavor and is incredibly filling. Pile a big scoop on top of some whole grains for an easy plant-based lunch or dinner bowl.

- 2 tablespoons extra-virgin olive oil
- 1 can (15.5 oz) chickpeas, drained and rinsed
- 2 cloves garlic, minced
- 1 teaspoon smoked paprika
- ½ teaspoon ground turmeric
- ¼ teaspoon salt, plus salt as needed
- 6 cups chopped stemmed kale
- ½ cup low-sodium vegetable broth

Warm the olive oil in a large frying pan over medium heat. Add the chickpeas and cook for 3 minutes, until the chickpeas begin to brown.

Add the garlic, paprika, turmeric, and ¼ teaspoon of salt and cook for 1 to 2 minutes longer, until the chickpeas are coated in the spice mixture. Add the kale and broth and cook for 5 to 7 minutes, until the kale has wilted and the broth has evaporated. Season to taste with salt.

Serve immediately or store in a sealed container in the fridge for up to 5 days.

PER SERVING: Calories: 230, Fat: 10g, Sat Fat: 1g, Sodium: 400mg, Carbohydrates: 28g, Dietary Fiber: 8g, Added Sugar: 0g, Protein: 9g, Vitamin D: 0mcg, Calcium: 88mg, Iron: 2mg, Potassium: 263mg

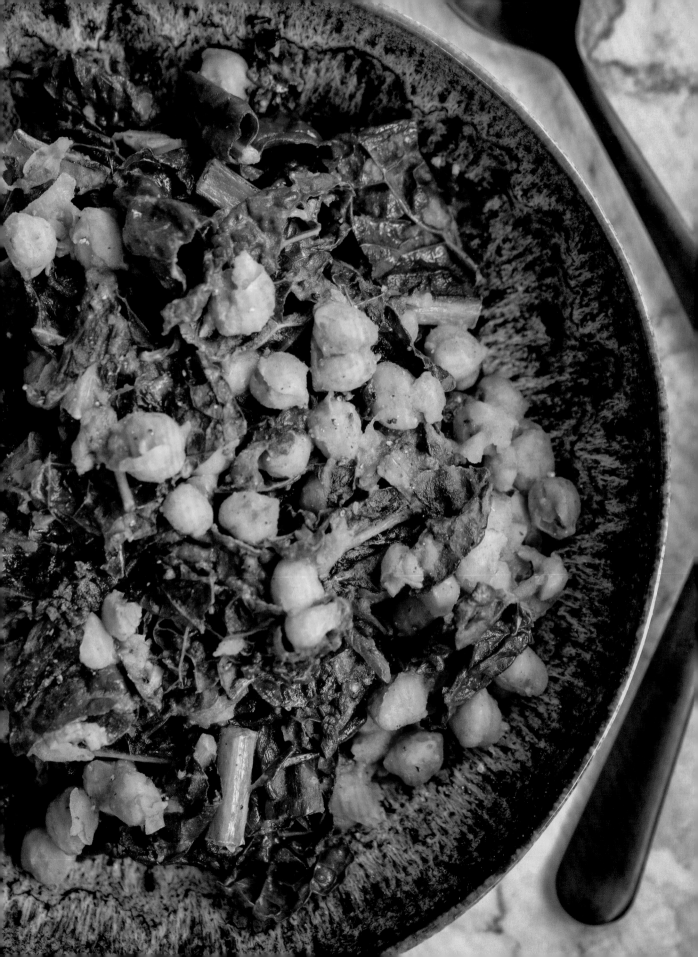

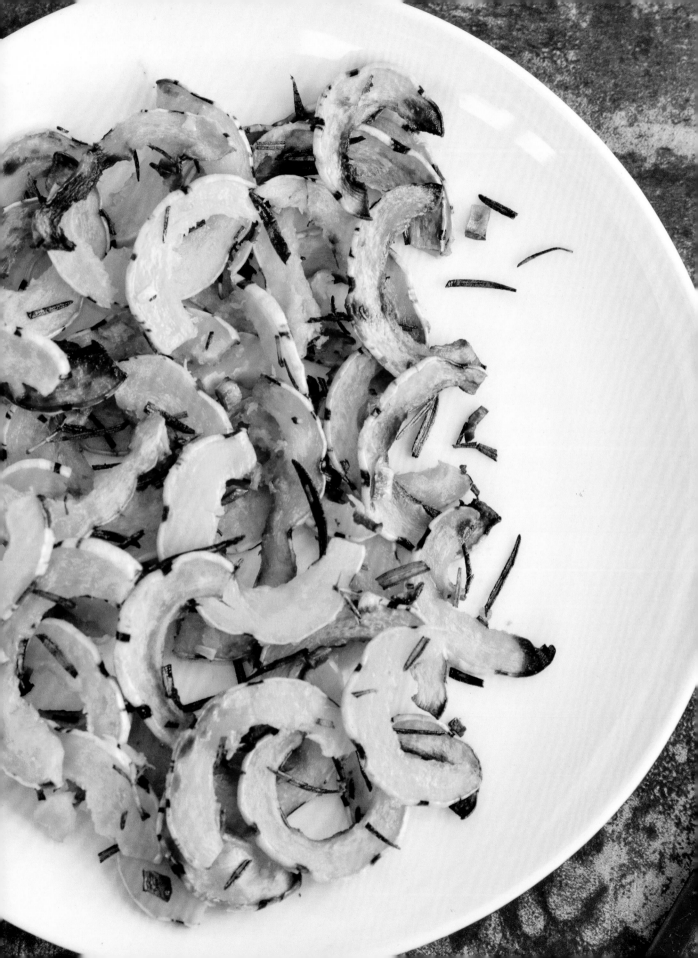

ROSEMARY ROASTED DELICATA SQUASH

MAKES 4 SERVINGS • PREP TIME: 10 MINUTES / COOK TIME: 30 MINUTES

Delicata squash is one of my fall and winter go-tos because you don't need to peel it before cooking. Unlike other types of squash, delicata has a thin peel that cooks up nicely and is easy to eat. Spice up the roasted squash with a pinch of fresh rosemary for an herbaceous side dish. Serve this alongside the Wild Rice and Mushroom Umami Burgers (page 90) for a starchy side.

2 small delicata squash, halved and seeded

2 tablespoons extra-virgin olive oil

2 tablespoons chopped stemmed fresh rosemary

4 cloves garlic, minced

¼ teaspoon salt

Preheat the oven to 400°F. Line a baking sheet with parchment paper.

Slice the squash into half-moons. You should have about 4 cups. Place them in a large bowl. Add the olive oil, rosemary, garlic, and salt. Toss well.

Transfer the seasoned squash to the prepared baking sheet. Bake for 30 minutes, until the edges are golden brown.

Serve immediately or store in a sealed container in the fridge for up to 5 days.

PER SERVING: Calories: 150, Fat: 7g, Sat Fat: 1g, Sodium: 150mg, Carbohydrates: 24g, Dietary Fiber: 3g, Added Sugar: 0g, Protein: 2g, Vitamin D: 0mcg, Calcium: 80mg, Iron: 2mg, Potassium: 767mg

VEGAN BUFFALO CAULIFLOWER BITES

MAKES 4 SERVINGS   •   PREP TIME: 10 MINUTES / COOK TIME: 35 MINUTES

You don't have to miss out on your favorite comfort foods when you follow a plant-based diet. These buffalo cauliflower bites are much healthier than chicken wings but still have the same spicy meaty taste. They're also baked, not fried, making them a healthier alternative for game day, a watch party, or a regular old spicy weeknight. The yogurt ranch (page 100) is a perfect dipping sauce.

1 head cauliflower, chopped into florets (6 cups)

1½ cups all-purpose flour

1 cup unsweetened almond milk

1 teaspoon salt

Cooking spray

½ cup cayenne pepper sauce, such as Frank's RedHot

2 tablespoons neutral oil (canola, vegetable, or grapeseed)

Preheat the oven to 375°F.

In three separate large bowls, individually place the cauliflower, flour, and almond milk. Add the salt to the flour bowl and mix well. Dip each piece of cauliflower into the bowl of almond milk, then dip it into the bowl with the flour mixture.

Once all pieces of cauliflower are coated, discard the leftover almond milk and the flour mixture.

Coat a large baking sheet with cooking spray and place each piece of dredged cauliflower on the prepared baking sheet. Spray the tops lightly with cooking spray. Bake for 35 minutes, until golden brown, then set aside to cool to the touch.

Meanwhile, in a small bowl, whisk together the cayenne pepper sauce and neutral oil.

Transfer the cooled cauliflower to a clean large bowl. Pour the hot sauce mixture on top and toss well to coat.

Garnish with parsley and serve immediately or store in a sealed container in the fridge for up to 3 days. Reheat in the oven at 350°F for 10 minutes when ready to serve.

PER SERVING: Calories: 220 calories, Fat: 8g, Sat Fat: 1g, Sodium: 1,360mg, Carbohydrates: 32g, Dietary Fiber: 4g, Added Sugar: 0g, Protein: 6g, Vitamin D: 0mcg, Calcium: 96mg, Iron: 1mg, Potassium: 534mg

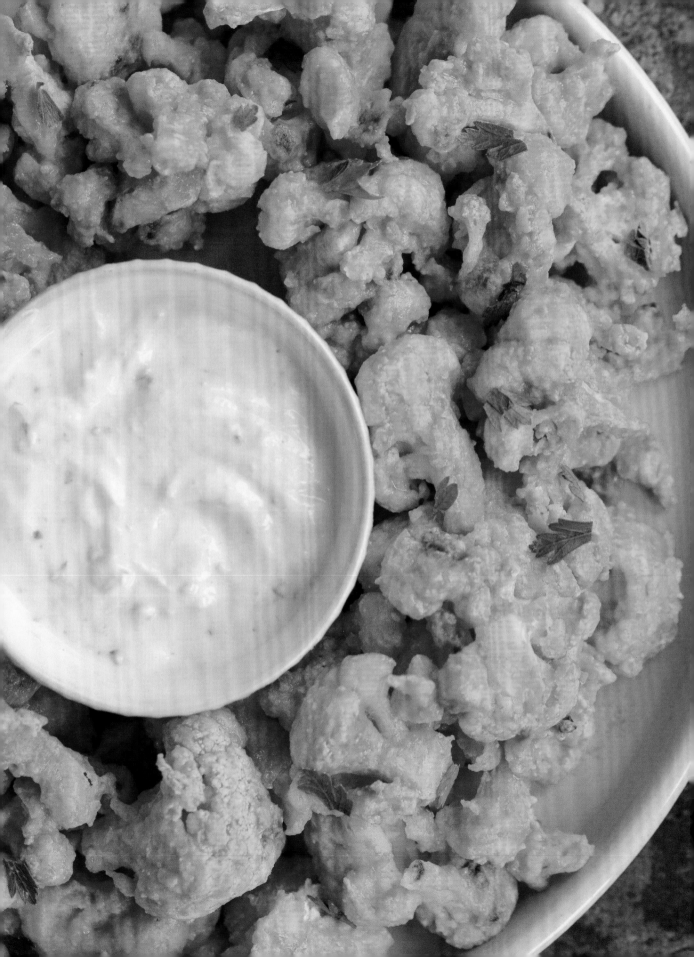

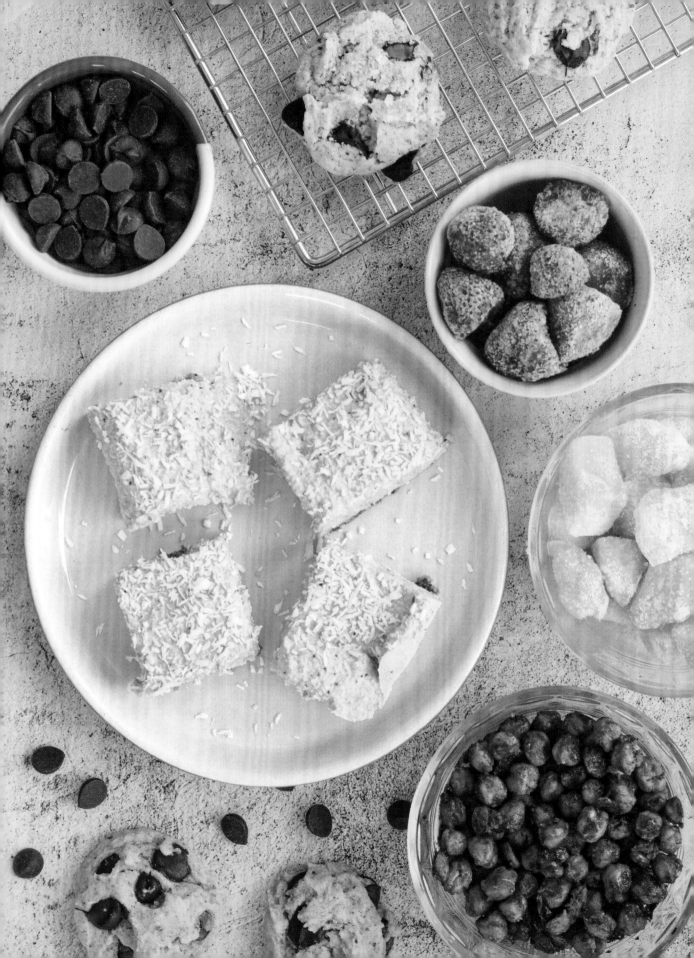

CHAPTER 7

EASY DESSERTS

For the busy athlete who doesn't want to spend hours baking a pie, these simple desserts will satisfy your sweet tooth. No fancy pastry skills required! And although these recipes are indulgent—hello Salted Tahini Chocolate Chip Cookies (page 130)—many are lower in added sugar and utilize fresh fruit. The Frozen Strawberry "Cheesecake" Bars (page 126) are a real plant-based showstopper that shows just how creamy blended cashews can be. Plus, these easy desserts provide nutrition and extra calories to an athlete's diet, which are much-needed treats for those training for a long-distance event.

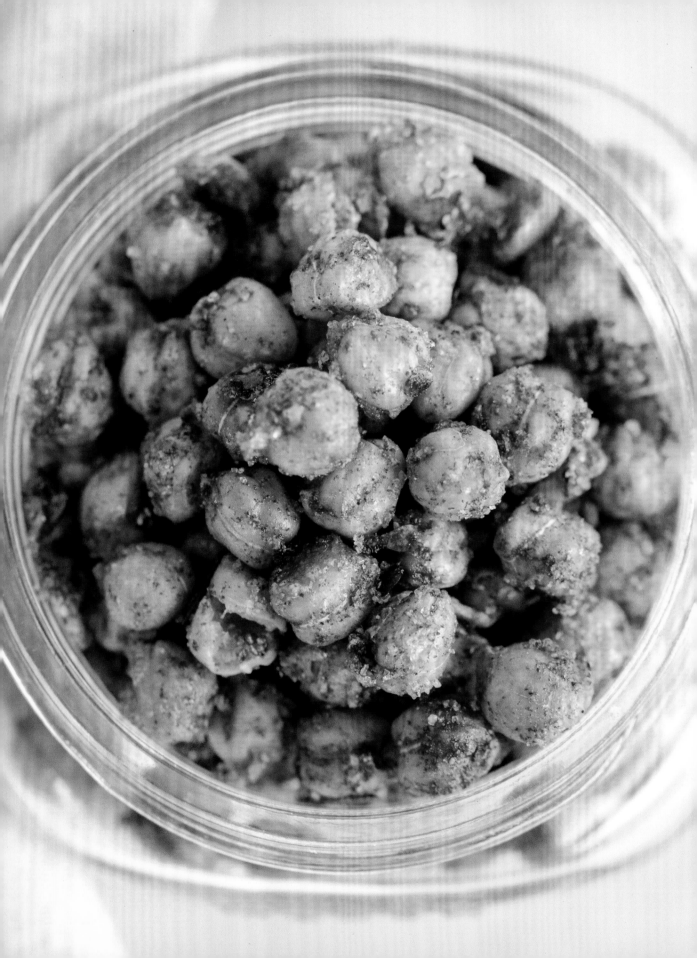

CINNAMON AND SUGAR ROASTED CHICKPEAS

MAKES 6 SERVINGS • **PREP TIME: 5 MINUTES / COOK TIME: 40 MINUTES**

This dish reminds me of a certain cinnamon and sugar–coated breakfast cereal. It brings me back to my childhood but in a much healthier way. These sweet legumes are baked in the oven and have just a touch of sugar. For intense training days, add this dessert with a healthy protein twist to your recovery routine for a nice, sweet treat.

2 cans (15.5 oz) chickpeas, drained and rinsed

2 tablespoons neutral oil (canola, vegetable, or grapeseed)

3 tablespoons sugar

2 teaspoons ground cinnamon

Preheat the oven to 400°F.

Place the chickpeas on a flat surface and pat dry with a towel. Place the chickpeas on a baking sheet and bake for 15 minutes.

Remove the chickpeas from the oven and let them cool slightly. Place in a large bowl and add the neutral oil, sugar, and cinnamon. Toss the chickpeas to coat.

Place the chickpeas back on the baking sheet and bake for 25 minutes longer, until crispy.

Serve immediately or store in an open container at room temperature for up to 3 days. The chickpeas may get slightly soft when stored, but the taste remains the same.

PER SERVING: Calories: 300, Fat: 12g, Sat Fat: 1g, Sodium: 470mg, Carbohydrates: 61g, Dietary Fiber: 15g, Added Sugar: 9g, Protein: 16g, Vitamin D: 0mcg, Calcium: 108mg, Iron: 2mg, Potassium: 245mg

WATERMELON SORBET

MAKES 4 SERVINGS • PREP TIME: 5 MINUTES

There's really nothing better on a hot summer day than frozen watermelon, and you'll be shocked at how easy it is to make this homemade sorbet. Fruit combines with sweetener and a squeeze of lemon juice to make a delightful frozen treat. As an added bonus, watermelon contains l-citrulline, a compound that increases blood flow and may improve athletic performance.

2 cups frozen watermelon

2 tablespoons maple syrup or honey

2 tablespoons fresh lemon juice

In a blender or food processor, combine the watermelon, maple syrup, and lemon juice. Process until smooth.

Serve immediately or store in a sealed container in the freezer for up to 1 month.

PER SERVING: Calories: 50, Fat: 0g, Sat Fat: 0g, Sodium: 0mg, Carbohydrates: 13g, Dietary Fiber: 0g, Added Sugar: 6g, Protein: 0g, Vitamin D: 0mcg, Calcium: 16mg, Iron: 0mg, Potassium: 114mg

Fun Facts

Want to switch up your sorbet flavor? Use other fresh melons, like honeydew or cantaloupe, in place of the watermelon. Other summer fruit, like pitted cherries or peeled peaches or plums, also work well in a sorbet.

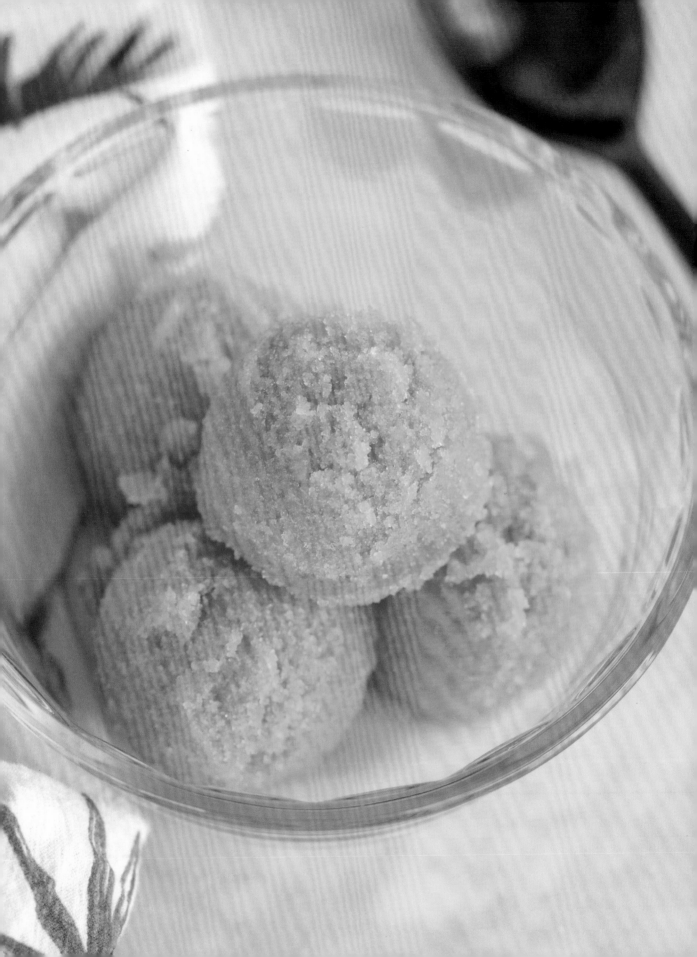

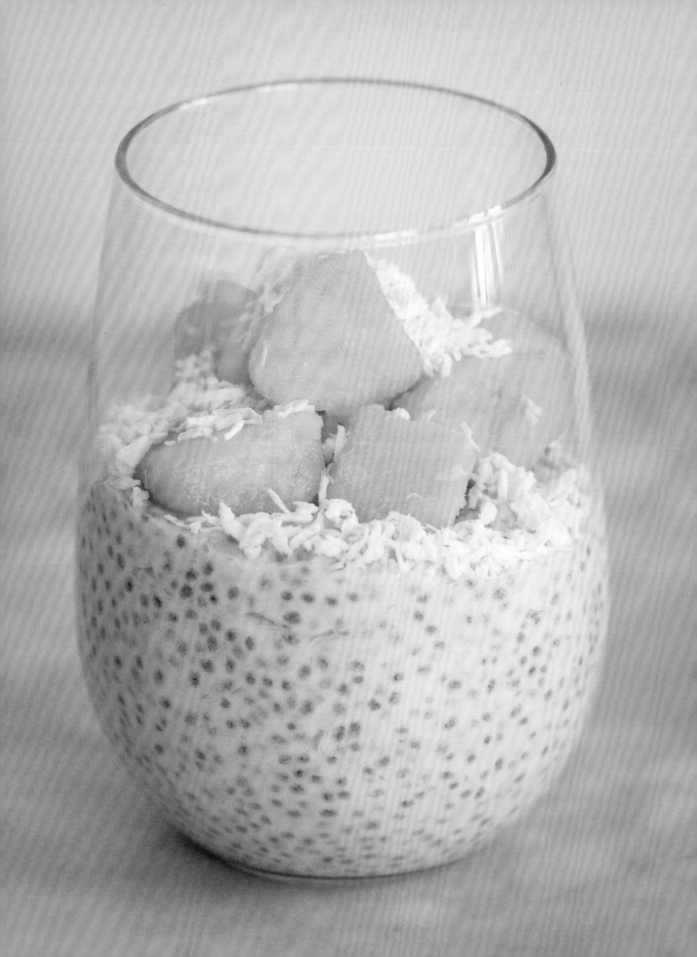

TROPICAL CHIA SEED PUDDING

MAKES 4 SERVINGS • PREP TIME: 5 MINUTES, PLUS 2 HOURS TO CHILL

This pudding tastes just like a piña colada and makes the perfect light dessert. Both pineapple and mango are loaded with vitamin C, which helps with immune system function, as well as potassium, which plays a role in electrolyte balance. Sweetened with just fruit, this dessert has zero added sugar. The mixture of coconut milk and chia seeds creates a luxurious creamy texture that you're going to want to eat on repeat.

2 cups coconut milk

2 cups frozen pineapple

2 cups frozen mango

2 cups unsweetened almond milk

½ cup chia seeds

Shredded coconut, for serving

Additional fruit, for serving

In a blender, combine the coconut milk, pineapple, mango, and almond milk. Blend until smooth.

Place the mixture in a large mason jar or other lidded container. Add the chia seeds, stir well, and refrigerate for at least 2 hours, until the mixture becomes thick.

Top with shredded coconut and fruit and serve immediately or store in a sealed container in the fridge for up to 5 days.

PER SERVING: Calories: 250, Fat: 13g, Sat Fat: 3.5g, Sodium: 125mg, Carbohydrates: 31g, Dietary Fiber: 8g, Added Sugar: 0g, Protein: 6g, Vitamin D: 3mcg, Calcium: 559mg, Iron: 2mg, Potassium: 489mg

BAKED PEARS WITH APPLE CIDER GLAZE

MAKES 4 SERVINGS • PREP TIME: 5 MINUTES / COOK TIME: 1 HOUR

This incredibly easy dessert impresses everyone who eats it. Baking pears with a touch of maple syrup and cinnamon brings out their inherent sweet flavor. Drizzle the pears with a simple apple cider glaze that is equal parts syrupy and savory. For added texture, throw some chopped nuts on top. Use a fork and knife to eat the whole pear, since most of the heart healthy fiber is in the peel.

4 pears, halved

2 tablespoons maple syrup

1½ teaspoons ground cinnamon, divided

1 cup apple cider or apple juice

½ cup powdered sugar

2 tablespoons unsalted butter or vegan butter

Pinch salt

Chopped nuts, for serving (optional)

Preheat the oven to 350°F.

Using a melon baller or small spoon, scoop the seeds out of the pears and discard.

In a small bowl, combine the maple syrup and 1 teaspoon of cinnamon, stirring well.

Place the pears on a baking sheet and drizzle the maple syrup mixture evenly over the pears. Bake for 1 hour, until the pears are fork-tender.

Meanwhile, in a small pot over high heat, bring the apple cider to a boil. Reduce the heat to low and simmer for 10 minutes. Add the powdered sugar, butter, remaining ½ teaspoon of cinnamon, and the salt and simmer for 5 minutes longer, until the mixture thickens.

Top the pears with chopped nuts, if using, then drizzle the apple cider glaze on top. Serve immediately.

PER SERVING: Calories: 270, Fat: 6g, Sat Fat: 3.5g, Sodium: 200mg, Carbohydrates: 57g, Dietary Fiber: 6g, Added Sugar: 21g, Protein: 1g, Vitamin D: 0mcg, Calcium: 43mg, Iron: 0mg, Potassium: 296mg

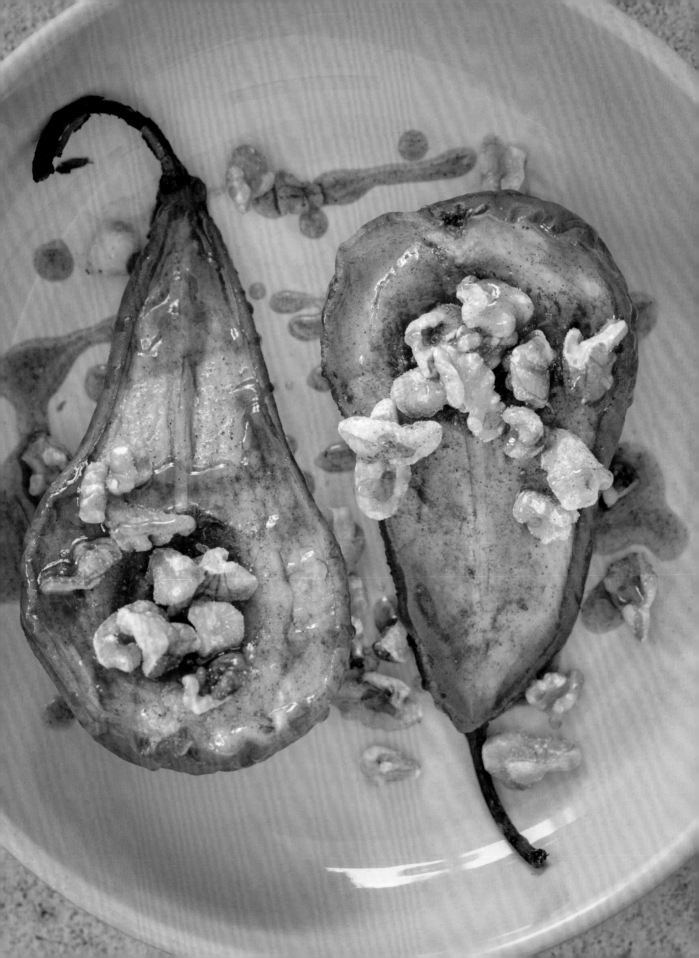

FROZEN STRAWBERRY "CHEESECAKE" BARS

MAKES 12 SERVINGS • PREP TIME: 15 MINUTES, PLUS OVERNIGHT TO SOAK AND 2 HOURS TO FREEZE

You won't miss the cheese in these raw frozen "cheesecake" bars. Made with soaked cashews, coconut milk, and strawberries, these creamy bars will satisfy your plant-based sweet tooth. And the best part is that there's no baking required! Eat them straight out of the freezer on a hot day, or let them sit out for 5 to 10 minutes to thaw.

FOR THE CRUST

1 cup dates, pitted

1 cup raw unsalted almonds

2 tablespoons unsweetened coconut flakes

1 teaspoon vanilla extract

½ teaspoon ground cinnamon

2 tablespoons water

FOR THE FILLING

2 cups raw unsalted cashews, soaked in water overnight (see tip)

½ cup coconut milk

3 tablespoons maple syrup

¼ cup fresh lemon juice

2 teaspoons vanilla extract

1 cup strawberries, stemmed

Sliced strawberries, for topping (optional)

Shredded coconut, for topping (optional)

To make the crust, in a food processor, combine the dates, almonds, coconut flakes, vanilla, cinnamon, and water. Blend until a well-combined mixture forms. It should be sticky to the touch. Line an 8-inch square pan with parchment paper. Press the mixture evenly into the prepared pan. Place in the fridge while preparing the filling.

Meanwhile, make the filling. In a food processor, puree the cashews, coconut milk, maple syrup, lemon juice, and vanilla until the mixture is smooth and creamy.

Pour half of the filling mixture into the crust. Leave the other half of the filling mixture in the food processor. Add the stemmed strawberries and process until well combined. Spread the strawberry layer over the plain layer.

Top with the sliced strawberries, if using, and shredded coconut, if using. Place the pan in the freezer for at least 2 hours before slicing into bars.

Transfer to a sealed container and store in the freezer for up to 1 month.

PER SERVING: Calories: 300, Fat: 20g, Sat Fat: 4g, Sodium: 10mg, Carbohydrates: 27g, Dietary Fiber: 4g, Added Sugar: 3g, Protein: 6g, Vitamin D: 0mcg, Calcium: 90mg, Iron: 44mg, Potassium: 261mg

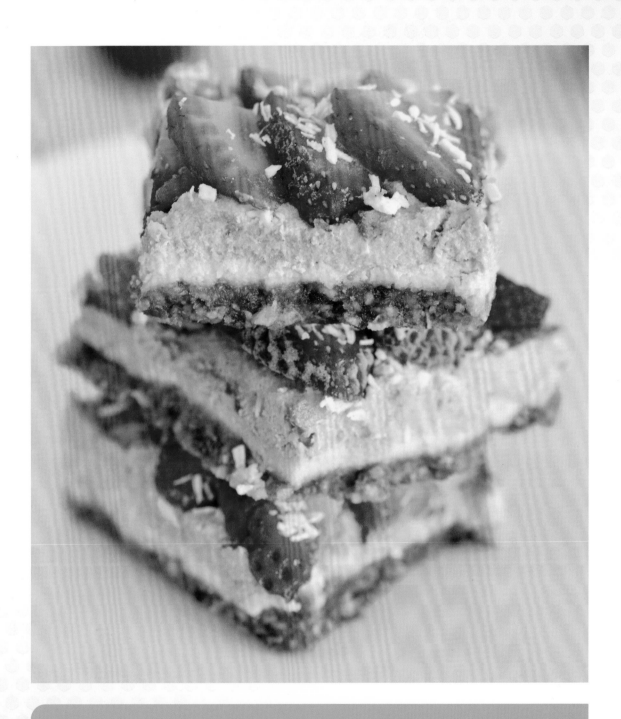

Tip: Soak cashews in water overnight. Drain the liquid before using. If you don't have time to soak the cashews overnight, pour boiling water over the cashews and let them sit in the water for 1 hour. Drain the water and use the soaked cashews.

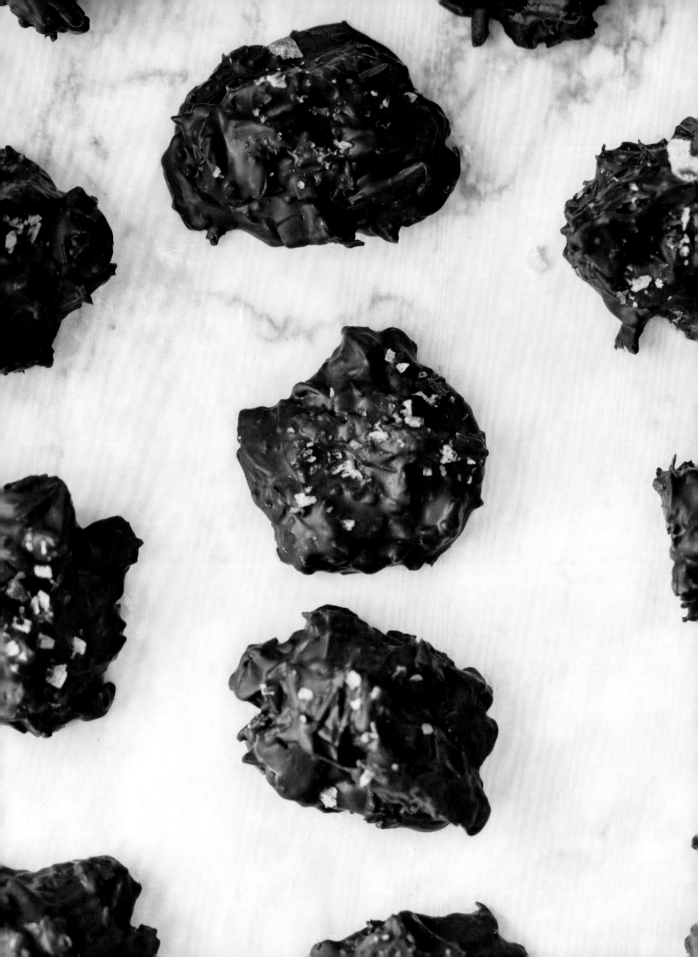

DARK CHOCOLATE AND CHERRY CLUSTERS

MAKES 6 SERVINGS • PREP TIME: 5 MINUTES, PLUS 1 HOUR TO CHILL / COOK TIME: 5 MINUTES

Calling all chocolate lovers! These chocolate clusters have a variety of flavors and textures in every bite. With four simple ingredients—dark chocolate, dried cherries, shredded coconut, and sliced almonds—these bites are rich, crunchy, and sweet. They are topped with a dash of coarse sea salt to bring out the flavor of the chocolate. All you need is a microwave and a fridge to make this simple chocolate-forward dessert.

1 cup dairy-free dark chocolate chips

¼ cup dried cherries, chopped

¼ cup shredded coconut

¼ cup unsalted toasted almonds

⅛ teaspoon coarse salt

In a large microwave safe bowl, microwave the chocolate on high power for 1 minute. Stir with a spatula and microwave for 30 seconds longer. Repeat this process 2 or 3 more times, making sure to thoroughly stir the chocolate after each heating, until the chocolate is melted.

Add the cherries, coconut, and almonds to the bowl. Stir well until all the ingredients are coated in chocolate.

Line a cutting board with parchment paper. Using a tablespoon, drop a cluster of the chocolate mixture onto the cutting board until all the chocolate is used.

Evenly sprinkle the salt over the chocolate clusters. Refrigerate for 1 hour, until set. Serve immediately or store in a sealed container in the fridge for up to 7 days.

PER SERVING: Calories: 120, Fat: 6g, Sat Fat: 3g, Sodium: 55mg, Carbohydrates: 18g, Dietary Fiber: 2g, Added Sugar: 13g, Protein: 2g, Vitamin D: 0mcg, Calcium: 13mg, Iron: 1mg, Potassium: 131mg

SALTED TAHINI CHOCOLATE CHIP COOKIES

MAKES 8 COOKIES • **PREP TIME: 5 MINUTES / COOK TIME: 15 MINUTES**

Tahini stands in for butter in these decadent chocolate chip cookies, creating a bite-size dessert that is nutty and rich. These cookies are crisp on the outside and soft on the inside. For a completely plant-based version, use flax eggs (see tip). The sprinkle of salt on top brings together the sweet and nutty flavors. You'll never want to eat a chocolate chip cookie without tahini again!

Cooking spray

½ cup tahini

½ cup plus 2 tablespoons sugar

2 large eggs or 2 flax eggs (see tip)

¼ cup neutral oil (canola, vegetable, or grapeseed)

1 tablespoon cold water

1 teaspoon vanilla extract

1 cup all-purpose flour

1 teaspoon baking powder

¼ teaspoon fine salt

½ cup semisweet chocolate chips

¼ teaspoon coarse sea salt or flaky salt

Preheat the oven to 350°F. Coat a baking sheet with cooking spray.

In a large bowl, combine the tahini and sugar. Using an electric mixer, beat until well combined. With the mixer going, add the eggs, neutral oil, water, and vanilla and continue to beat. Add the flour, baking powder, and fine salt, beating until well combined.

Turn off the mixer and add the chocolate chips. Use a spoon to evenly mix them into the batter.

Use a cookie dough scoop or a tablespoon to scoop out cookies onto the prepared baking sheet. Sprinkle a few drops of coarse salt on top of each cookie. Bake for 12 to 15 minutes, until the edges are golden brown.

Eat immediately or store in a sealed container at room temperature for up to 5 days or in the freezer for up to 1 month. When ready to eat, microwave for 30 seconds.

PER SERVING (2 COOKIES): Calories: 340, Fat: 19g, Sat Fat: 4g, Sodium: 130mg, Carbohydrates: 38g, Dietary Fiber: 2g, Added Sugar: 21g, Protein: 6g, Vitamin D: 0mcg, Calcium: 108mg, Iron: 1mg, Potassium: 140mg

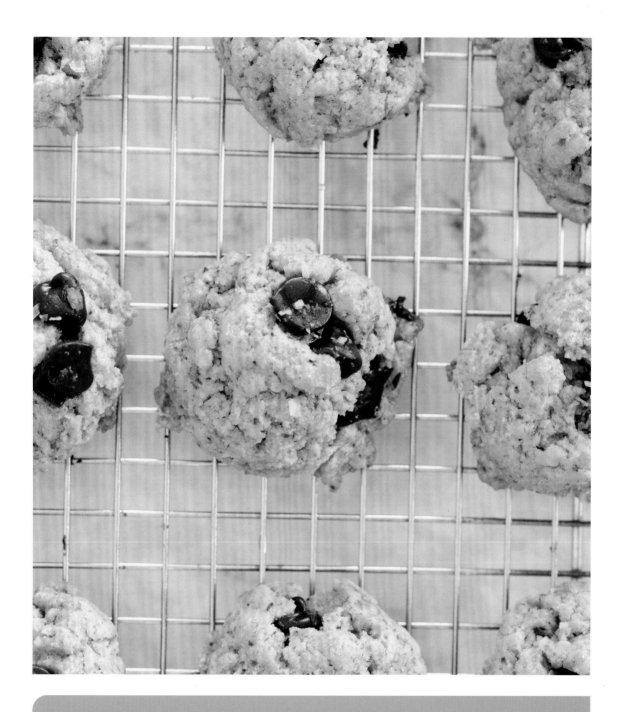

Vegan Tip: To make a flax egg, combine 1 tablespoon of flax meal with 3 tablespoons of warm water. Let it sit for at least 5 minutes, until the mixture thickens slightly.

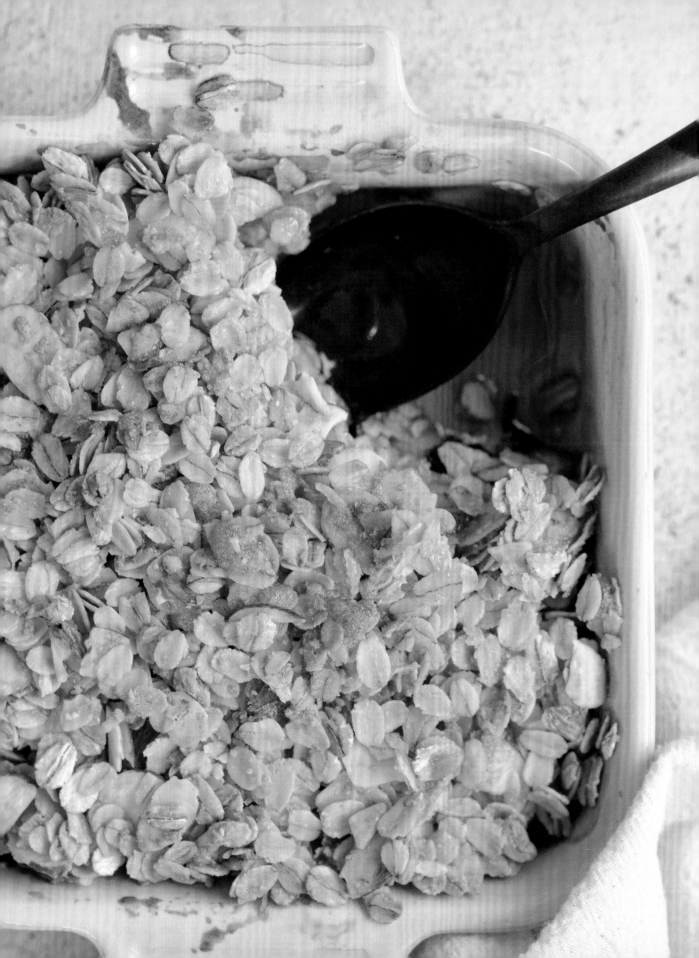

PLUM CRISP

MAKES 6 SERVINGS • **PREP TIME: 5 MINUTES / COOK TIME: 35 MINUTES**

A crisp is traditionally fruit covered with an oat, flour, and butter topping, which although delicious, isn't the healthiest of desserts. This revised version omits the flour and butter and lets the natural sugar from the fruit shine. Topped with a mixture of oats, almonds, and a little bit of sugar, this plum crisp is just as good as any other crisp out there.

Cooking spray

2 cups rolled oats

1 cup sliced raw unsalted almonds

¼ cup neutral oil (canola, vegetable, or grapeseed)

¼ cup dark brown sugar

¼ cup maple syrup

8 plums, pitted and chopped

Preheat the oven to 350°F. Coat an 8-inch square casserole dish with cooking spray.

In a large bowl, combine the oats, almonds, neutral oil, brown sugar, and maple syrup. Stir until well combined.

Place the plums in the prepared dish. Top with the oat mixture. Bake for 30 to 35 minutes, until the oats are golden brown.

Serve immediately or place a lid on the casserole dish and store in the fridge for up to 3 days.

PER SERVING: Calories: 410, Fat: 22g, Sat Fat: 1.5g, Sodium: 0mg, Carbohydrates: 48g, Dietary Fiber: 7g, Added Sugar: 16g, Protein: 9g, Vitamin D: 0mcg, Calcium: 72mg, Iron: 2mg, Potassium: 166mg

Fun Facts

Did you know that frozen fruits or veggies are nutritionally identical to fresh? They are frozen at the peak of ripeness, locking in all the amazing nutrients.

LEMON CAKE

MAKES 8 SERVINGS • PREP TIME: 5 MINUTES / COOK TIME: 25 MINUTES

Whip up this light and moist cake for the lemon lover in your life. The coconut milk is the perfect replacement for eggs in this recipe. It helps create a cake that is both light and moist at the same time. The cake tastes great on its own, but the glaze adds a hint more sweetness and lemon flavor. Top it off with a dash of lemon zest to really bring that lemon flavor home.

FOR THE CAKE

Cooking spray

2 cups all-purpose flour

½ cup granulated sugar

1 tablespoon baking powder

⅛ teaspoon fine salt

1 cup coconut milk

¼ cup neutral oil (canola, vegetable, or grapeseed)

¼ cup fresh lemon juice

2 teaspoons vanilla extract

1 teaspoon grated lemon zest

FOR THE GLAZE

⅓ cup powdered sugar

1 tablespoon fresh lemon juice

1 tablespoon milk

Preheat the oven to 350°F. Coat an 8-inch square baking pan with cooking spray.

To make the cake, in a large bowl, combine the flour, granulated sugar, baking powder, and salt. In a separate large bowl, combine the coconut milk, neutral oil, lemon juice, vanilla, and lemon zest. Whisk until the liquid ingredients are well combined. Pour the coconut milk mixture into the flour mixture and use a spatula to stir until all the ingredients are combined.

Pour the batter in the prepared pan. Bake for 25 minutes, until the edges of the cake are golden brown.

Meanwhile, make the glaze. In a small bowl, whisk together the powdered sugar, lemon juice, and milk until well combined and all the sugar clumps are dissolved.

Let the cake cool to the touch, then pour the glaze on top.

Serve immediately or store in a sealed container in the fridge for up to 5 days or in the freezer for up to 1 month. Microwave frozen cake slices for 30 seconds when ready to eat.

PER SERVING: Calories: 260, Fat: 8g, Sat Fat: 1g, Sodium: 35mg, Carbohydrates: 44g, Dietary Fiber: 1g, Added Sugar: 18g, Protein: 3g, Vitamin D: 0mcg, Calcium: 291mg, Iron: 1mg, Potassium: 51mg

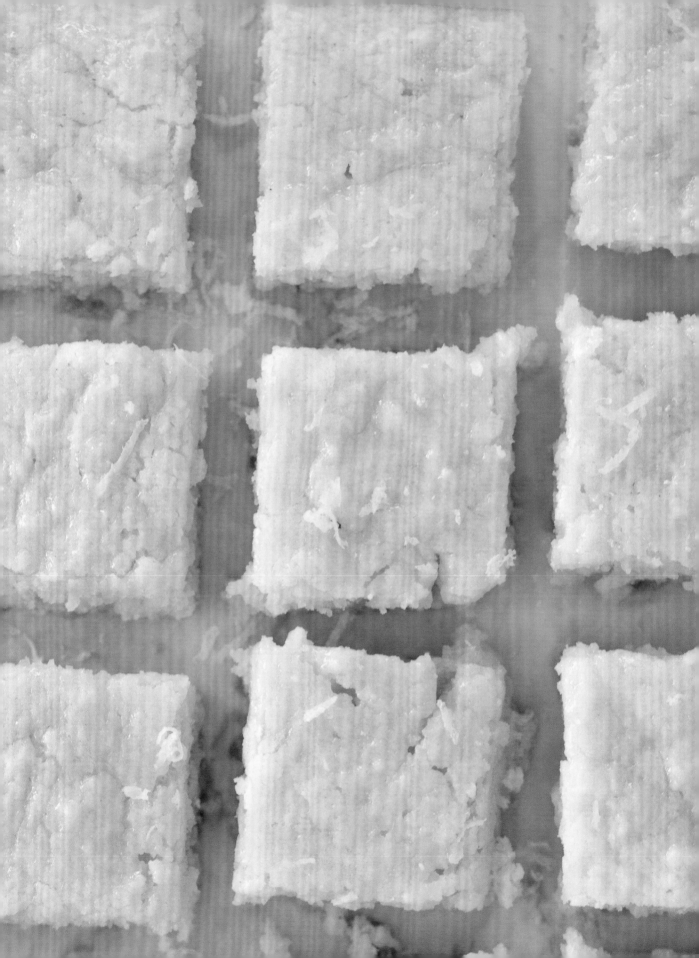

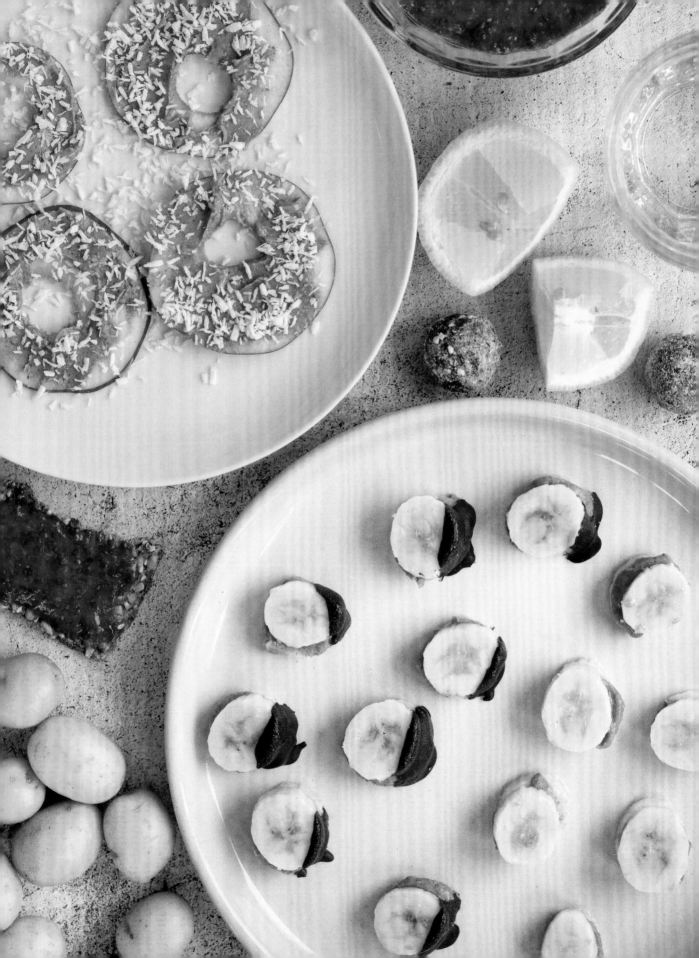

CHAPTER 8

WORKOUT FUEL

For endurance athletes who work out for longer than 60 minutes, fueling during exercise is necessary to maintain energy levels. While there are a ton of sports nutrition products on the market, sometimes it's easier and healthier to whip up your own workout fuel. This chapter contains a mixture of homemade sports drinks and easy-to-digest snacks that are portable and provide quick energy during a workout. If you're like me and don't love the taste of a sports drink, try the Salted Watermelon Sports Drink (page 138) or the Lemon-Lime Sports Drink (page 140). If bananas are more your thing, the Frozen Peanut Butter Banana Bites (page 142) are easy to eat and provide much needed electrolytes, such as potassium and sodium, as well as quick-acting carbs. And for those who are sick of sweet sports nutrition products, try the simple Potato Cakes (page 149) and stuff them in your pack during a long bout of endurance activity.

SALTED WATERMELON SPORTS DRINK

MAKES 2 SERVINGS • **PREP TIME: 5 MINUTES**

Sports drinks should have sugar to provide that extra boost you need for an intense workout, but they don't need to be overly sweet. The combination of watermelon, coconut water, and salt creates a well-balanced sports beverage that has sugar, fluid, and electrolytes—all the ingredients you need to power you through a tough training session. Not to mention, this homemade sports drink has no unnecessary color or flavor additives, unlike many bottled versions.

¾ cup watermelon juice or 1 cup fresh watermelon, blended

16 ounces coconut water

1 teaspoon honey or maple syrup

¼ teaspoon salt

In a mason jar or other jar with a lid, combine the watermelon juice, coconut water, honey, and salt. Close tightly and shake well.

Serve immediately or store in the fridge for up to 5 days.

PER SERVING: Calories: 100, Fat: 0g, Sat Fat: 0g, Sodium: 330mg, Carbohydrates: 25g, Dietary Fiber: 0g, Added Sugar: 3g, Protein: 1g, Vitamin D: 0mcg, Calcium: 52mg, Iron: 0mg, Potassium: 644mg

Fun Facts

Sports drink recipes are simple because they need to be easy to make and digest. But if your tastebuds are getting a bit bored, add a squeeze of lime juice or a sprig of fresh mint to this drink to spice it up.

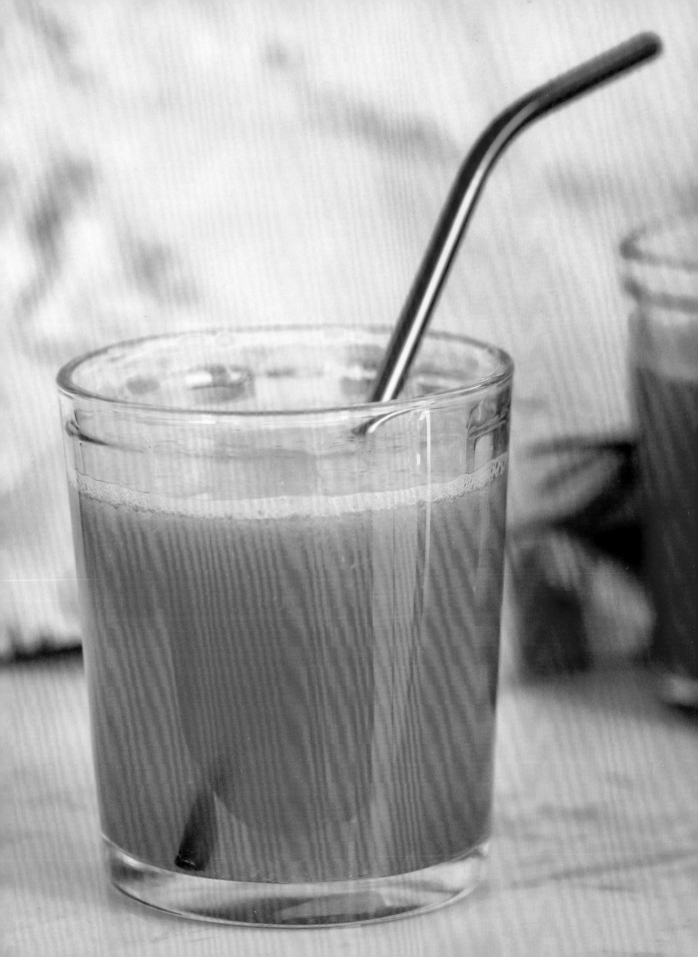

LEMON-LIME SPORTS DRINK

MAKES 2 SERVINGS • **PREP TIME: 5 MINUTES**

If your go-to sports drink is the standard lemon-lime flavor, you're going to love this homemade version. Made with actual lemon and lime juice and mixed with coconut water, sweetener, and salt, this sports drink stacks up to any of the ones on store shelves. Plus, it takes only minutes to make, and it won't put a dent in your wallet during training season.

16 ounces coconut water

2 tablespoons fresh lime juice

2 tablespoons fresh lemon juice

2 teaspoons honey or maple syrup

¼ teaspoon salt

In a mason jar or other jar with a lid, combine the coconut water, lime juice, lemon juice, honey, and salt. Close tightly and shake well.

Serve immediately or store in the fridge for up to 5 days.

PER SERVING: Calories: 90, Fat: 0g, Sat Fat: 0g, Sodium: 330mg, Carbohydrates: 24g, Dietary Fiber: 0g, Added Sugar: 6g, Protein: 1g, Vitamin D: 0mcg, Calcium: 49mg, Iron: 0mg, Potassium: 579mg

Fun Facts

Research suggests that rinsing your mouth with a sports drink and spitting it out may be as good as drinking it. When carbohydrates come into contact with the mouth, your brain and central nervous system receive perceptions of well-being while exercising.

HOMEMADE STRAWBERRY CHIA JAM

MAKES 4 SERVINGS • PREP TIME: 5 MINUTES / COOK TIME: 10 MINUTES

One of my favorite things to eat during a workout is jam. It may sound simple, but the carbs in the jam give me plenty of energy to power through a workout without irritating my stomach. Although store-bought jams are super convenient, this strawberry jam has a little extra nutrition boost from the natural fruit, chia seeds, and maple syrup. You get not only carbs from the fruit and syrup but also an added protein and fiber boost from the chia seeds.

2 cups chopped strawberries

2 tablespoons chia seeds

2 tablespoons maple syrup

¼ cup water

In a small pot over high heat, combine the strawberries, chia seeds, maple syrup, and water. Bring to a boil, then reduce the heat to low and simmer for 10 minutes, until the liquid is absorbed. Remove from the heat.

Let the jam cool slightly, then transfer it to a food processor. Process until all the chunks are removed.

Divvy the jam into four lock-top plastic bags. When ready to eat, squeeze it out of the bag and directly into your mouth (like a sports gel). Store leftover jam in its bag in the fridge for up to 2 weeks.

PER SERVING: Calories: 80, Fat: 2.5g, Sat Fat: 0g, Sodium: 25mg, Carbohydrates: 15g, Dietary Fiber: 4g, Added Sugar: 6g, Protein: 2g, Vitamin D: 0mcg, Calcium: 62mg, Iron: 1mg, Potassium: 131mg

FROZEN PEANUT BUTTER BANANA BITES

MAKES 2 SERVINGS • PREP TIME: 5 MINUTES, PLUS 1 HOUR TO FREEZE / COOK TIME: 5 MINUTES

Have you ever trained for an event in the heat of summer? Your hunger diminishes during a hot sweaty workout, even though you need the extra food. These frozen carb-rich snacks are easy to get down when you're hot, exhausted, and need a little extra fuel in your system. As a bonus, the potassium in the banana helps replenish the electrolytes lost in sweat. If you're feeling extra fancy, dip them in a dark-chocolate coating.

- 2 tablespoons salted peanut butter
- 2 bananas, cut into 1-inch slices
- 2 tablespoons dark chocolate chips (optional)

Line a baking sheet with parchment paper.

Spread the peanut butter on half of the banana slices and place another banana slice on top of each one, making mini sandwiches.

Place the chocolate, if using, in a small microwave-safe bowl and on high power microwave for 1 minute. Stir and microwave again for 30 seconds. Repeat until all the chocolate has melted and there are no visible chunks.

Dip each banana sandwich into the chocolate and place it on the prepared baking sheet. Freeze for at least 1 hour. Serve immediately and sprinkle with little rock salt (if desired). Store in a sealed container in the freezer for up to 1 month.

PER SERVING: Calories: 200, Fat: 8g, Sat Fat: 1g, Sodium: 70mg, Carbohydrates: 30g, Dietary Fiber: 4g, Added Sugar: 0g, Protein: 5g, Vitamin D: 0mcg, Calcium: 16mg, Iron: 1mg, Potassium: 522mg

Fun Facts

One medium banana has 100% the daily value of potassium, an electrolyte that helps with muscle contraction, nerve function, heart rate, and fluid balance. Moreover, potassium is one of the electrolytes lost in sweat.

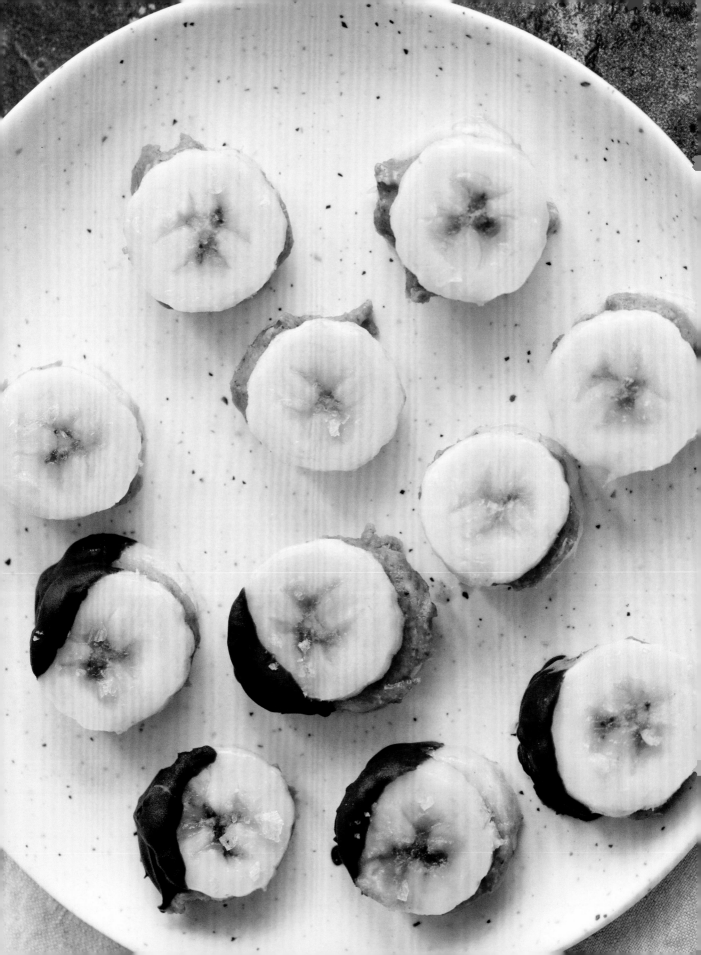

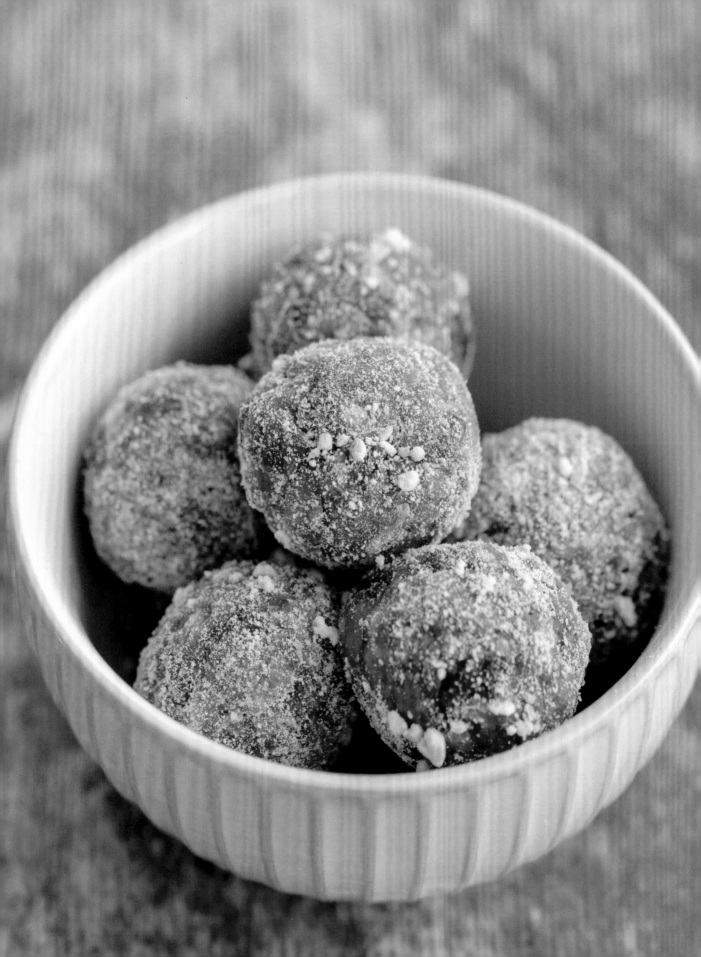

SWEET AND SALTY PRETZEL DATE BITES

MAKES 12 BITES • PREP TIME: 5 MINUTES, PLUS 1 HOUR TO CHILL

This combination of dates and pretzels is the perfect duo of salty and sweet. Made with three simple ingredients, these bites are held together with nut butter and are easy to pop in your mouth during a training session. The dates and pretzels provide carbs for quick-acting energy, while the nut butter offers protein to aid in postworkout muscle recovery.

¼ cup pretzels

1 cup pitted dates

2 tablespoons peanut butter

Line a baking sheet or plate with parchment paper.

In a food processor, process the pretzels into crumbs. Set aside in a small bowl.

Combine the dates and peanut butter in the food processor and process until crumbly. Using your hands, form the date mixture into 2- to 3-inch balls (about the size of a ping-pong ball).

Roll each ball in the pretzel crumbs and place on the prepared baking sheet. Refrigerate for about 1 hour. Serve immediately or store in a sealed container in the fridge for up to 7 days.

PER SERVING (2 BITES): Calories: 160, Fat: 3.5g, Sat Fat: 0.5g, Sodium: 370mg, Carbohydrates: 29g, Dietary Fiber: 1g, Added Sugar: 0g, Protein: 4g, Vitamin D: 0mcg, Calcium: 14mg, Iron: 1mg, Potassium: 136mg

APPLE RING SAMOAS

MAKES 2 SERVINGS • **PREP TIME: 10 MINUTES**

Named after the Girl Scout cookies that have caramel, chocolate, and coconut, this apple version is easy to prepare and digest, making it ideal workout fuel. Most caramel sauces are not plant-based because they contain milk. These plant-based cookies are made with cookie butter (from the speculoos cookie) for a similar taste. It's easy to spread and has a sweet taste the pairs well with apples. The sprinkle of shredded coconut on top adds an extra hint of sweetness.

2 tablespoons cookie butter

2 red apples, cored and cut crosswise into ½-inch-thick rings

2 teaspoons shredded coconut

Spread a thin layer of cookie butter on all the apple slices. Sprinkle with coconut.

Serve right away or store in a sealed container in the fridge for up to 3 days.

PER SERVING: Calories: 240, Fat: 8g, Sat Fat: 3.5g, Sodium: 15mg, Carbohydrates: 41g, Dietary Fiber: 5g, Added Sugar: 0g, Protein: 2g, Vitamin D: 0mcg, Calcium: 14mg, Iron: 0mg, Potassium: 240mg

Fun Facts

"An apple a day keeps the doctor away" may be true, since one apple is a good source of Vitamin C. Not to mention that the skin of the apple is packed with fiber. Many endurance athletes fuel with applesauce, since it's naturally sweet and easy to digest.

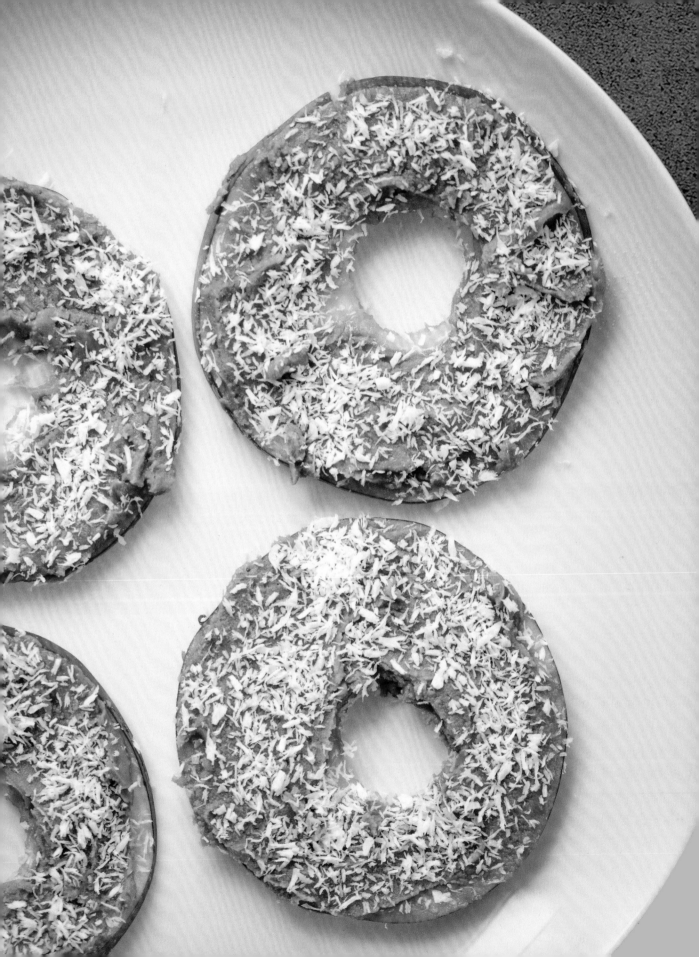

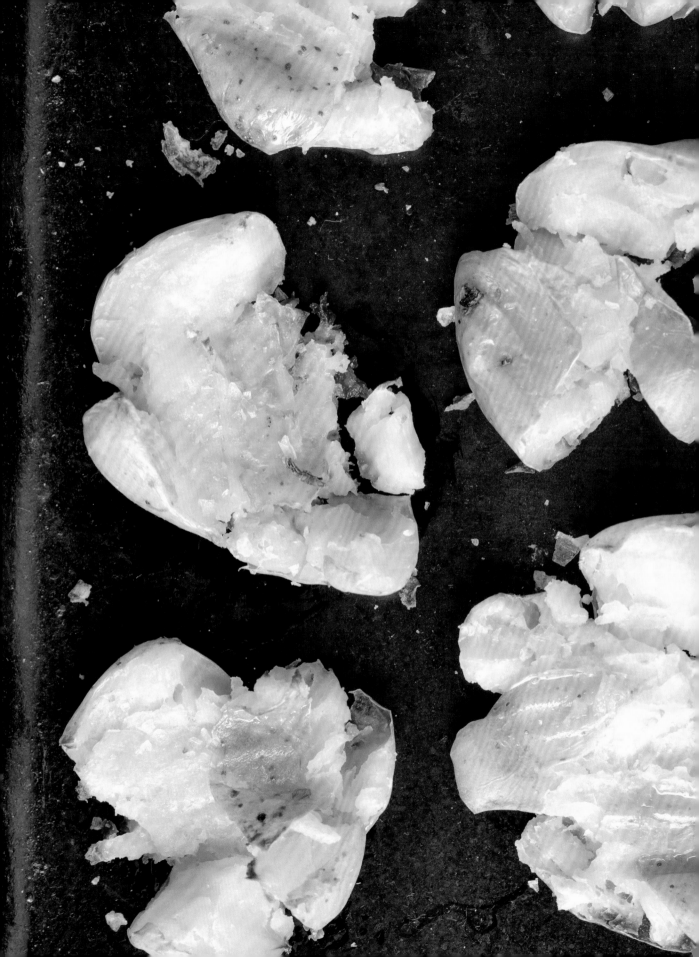

POTATO CAKES

MAKES 4 SERVINGS • **PREP TIME: 10 MINUTES / COOK TIME: 40 MINUTES**

For those who prefer savory over sweet (that's me!), these potato cakes are a great make-ahead carb that packs easily for midtraining fuel. The simple starch of the potato breaks down quickly to release energy into your bloodstream during activity. So, if you're sick of sweet sports products or just want to change things up, whip up a batch of these baby potato cakes.

¾ pound baby yellow potatoes

2 tablespoons extra-virgin olive oil

¼ teaspoon coarse salt

In a large pot over high heat, combine the potatoes with enough water to cover. Bring to a boil and cook for 20 minutes, until tender. Remove from the heat, drain the water from the pot, and let the potatoes cool slightly, about 5 minutes.

Preheat the oven to 400°F. Once the potatoes are cool enough to touch, place them on a baking sheet. Use a fork to press them down and mash them. Drizzle the olive oil on top and bake for 20 minutes, until golden brown. Sprinkle the potato cakes with salt.

Serve right away or store in a sealed container in the fridge for up to 5 days. Eat cold or microwave on high power for 1 minute to warm them up before packing.

PER SERVING: Calories: 120, Fat: 7g, Sat Fat: 1g, Sodium: 150mg, Carbohydrates: 15g, Dietary Fiber: 2g, Added Sugar: 0g, Protein: 2g, Vitamin D: 0mcg, Calcium: 62mg, Iron: 1mg, Potassium: 0mg

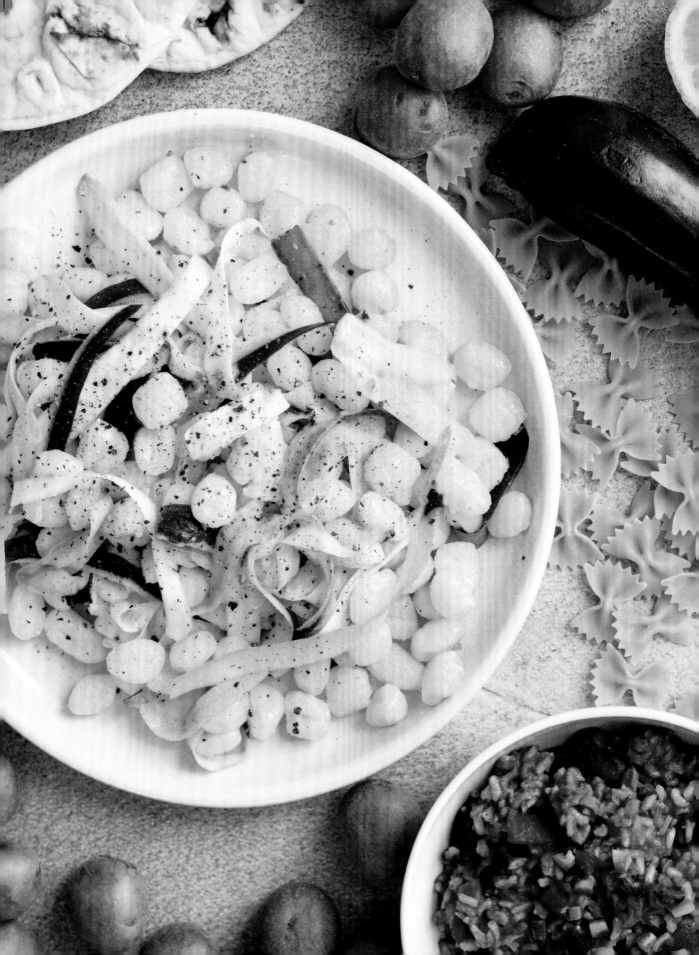

CHAPTER 9

CARB-LOADING STAPLES

If you're gearing up for a long-distance endurance event, you may want to carb load the week leading up to the race. Carb loading involves consuming around 80 percent of your calories from carbs, and doing so is more difficult than you might imagine. Usually, glycogen only lasts for about 30 minutes during exercise. The purpose of carb loading is to store up as much glycogen as possible to try to extend that 30-minute window. While carb loading, you'll want to eat foods that are easy to digest and won't wreak havoc on your gastrointestinal system during your upcoming event. These recipes include some of the highest carb foods that won't cause any stomach issues, such as pasta, rice, and potatoes.

CURRY COCONUT QUINOA WITH SPINACH

MAKES 4 SERVINGS • **PREP TIME: 5 MINUTES / COOK TIME: 15 MINUTES**

When I tell you that this recipe is ready in just 20 minutes flat, I'm not exaggerating. The only thing that needs to be prepped is the minced garlic. Otherwise, everything cooks in one pot and gives off this amazing coconut curry aroma. Simply simmer the quinoa, spices, coconut milk, and spinach in one pot and top with sliced almonds. This is one of my favorite carb-loading staples, but it also works well as a side dish or light lunch.

1 tablespoon extra-virgin olive oil

3 cloves garlic, minced

1 cup quinoa

¾ teaspoon curry powder

½ teaspoon ground turmeric

½ teaspoon salt, plus salt as needed

½ cup full-fat coconut milk

1½ cups water

2 cups packed spinach

¼ cup sliced raw unsalted almonds

Freshly ground black pepper

In a medium pot over medium heat, combine the olive oil and garlic. Cook for 2 minutes, until the garlic is golden brown. Add the quinoa, curry powder, turmeric, and ½ teaspoon of salt. Stir to combine.

Add the coconut milk, water, and spinach to the pot and bring to a boil. Cover, reduce the heat to low, and simmer for 15 minutes, until all the liquid is absorbed. Season to taste with salt and black pepper.

Divide the quinoa among four bowls and top each with 1 tablespoon of almonds. Store leftovers in a sealed container in the fridge for up to 7 days.

PER SERVING: Calories: 300, Fat: 16g, Sat Fat: 6g, Sodium: 310mg, Carbohydrates: 31g, Dietary Fiber: 5g, Added Sugar: 0g, Protein: 9g, Vitamin D: 0mcg, Calcium: 64mg, Iron: 4mg, Potassium: 390mg

Fun Facts

Turmeric is a potent antioxidant. Small studies indicate that supplementing with the active form of turmeric—called cumin—may improve postexercise recovery and help reduce muscle soreness.

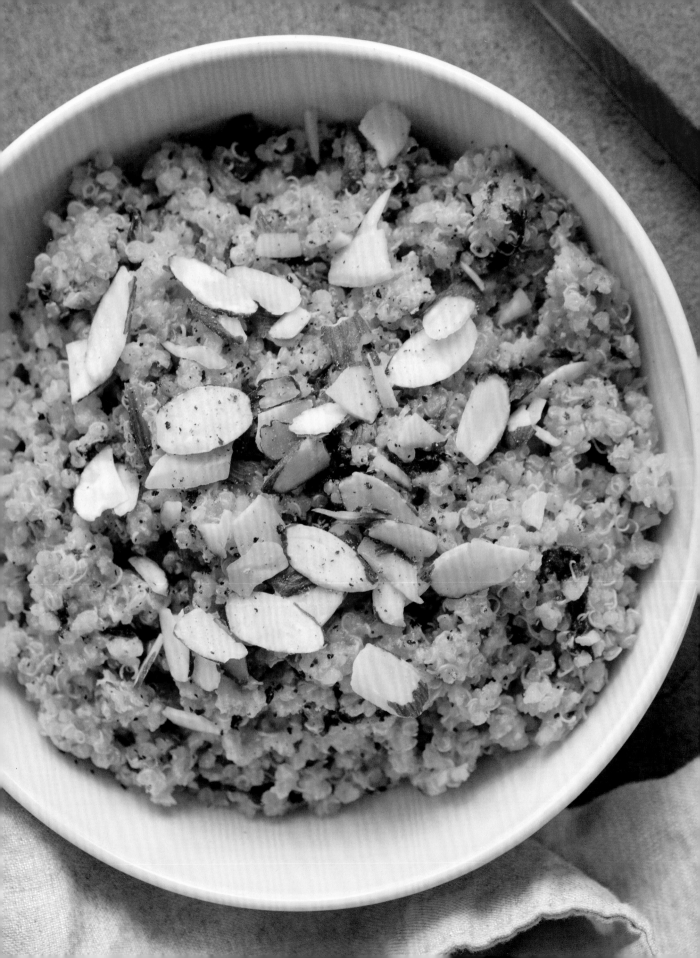

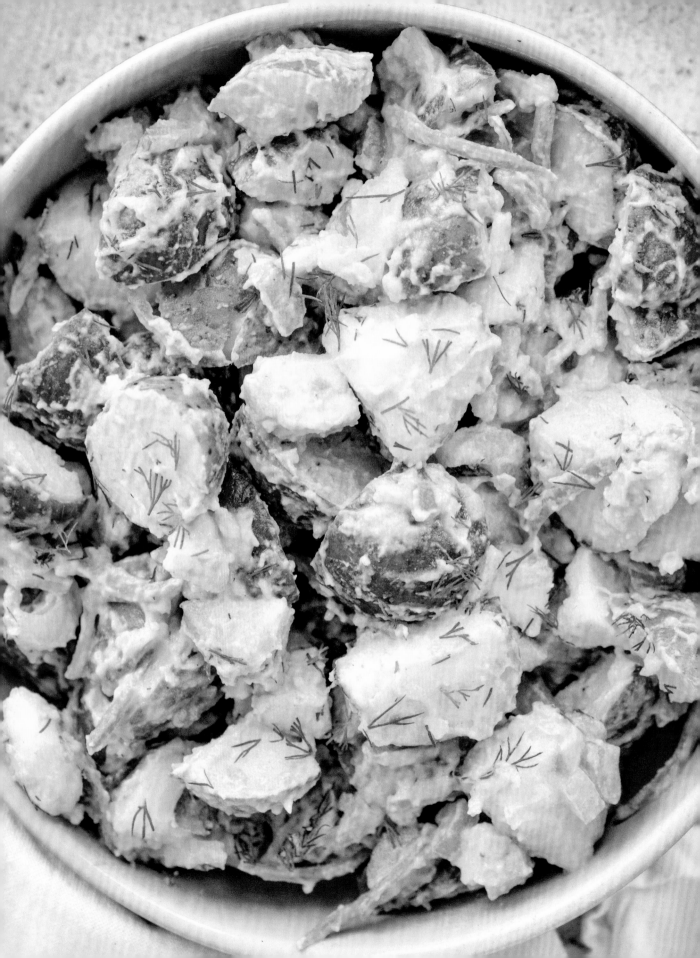

AVOCADO POTATO SALAD

MAKES 4 SERVINGS • PREP TIME: 5 MINUTES / COOK TIME: 10 MINUTES

Say goodbye to the potato salad covered in globs of mayo or other indistinguishable sauces. This recipe has just a touch of mayo, combined with creamy avocado, veggies, and herbs. Although carbs are a huge part of an athlete's diet, many endurance enthusiasts neglect healthy fats. Avocados are loaded with good-for-you monounsaturated fats, which help satisfy your hunger after an intense training session and contribute to brain and heart health.

I pound baby red potatoes, quartered

¼ cup mayonnaise or vegan mayonnaise

2 tablespoons Dijon mustard

I tablespoon apple cider vinegar

½ teaspoon salt, plus salt as needed

I avocado, pitted, peeled, and finely chopped

½ cup chopped celery

½ cup shredded carrots

1½ tablespoons chopped fresh dill

Freshly ground black pepper

Bring a large pot of salted water to a boil over high heat. Add the potatoes and cook for 10 minutes. Drain the water and set aside the potatoes.

In a small bowl, prepare the dressing by whisking together the mayonnaise, mustard, vinegar, and ½ teaspoon of salt.

Place the cooked potatoes, avocado, celery, carrots, and dill in a large bowl. Pour the dressing on top and mix well. Season to taste with salt and black pepper.

Serve immediately or store in a sealed contained in the fridge for up to 3 days. The avocado mixture will brown, but it's still safe to eat.

PER SERVING: Calories: 240, Fat: 16g, Sat Fat: 2.5g, Sodium: 540mg, Carbohydrates: 22g, Dietary Fiber: 5g, Added Sugar: 0g, Protein: 3g, Vitamin D: 0mcg, Calcium: 24mg, Iron: Img, Potassium: 728mg

SMOKY RICE AND BEANS

MAKES 4 SERVINGS • **PREP TIME: 5 MINUTES / COOK TIME: 35 MINUTES**

Rice and beans is a plant-based staple, especially for those looking to up their carb game. This recipe is one of my favorite types: a one-pot wonder that has tons of flavor. It takes traditional rice and beans up a notch with smoked paprika and fire-roasted tomatoes, both of which add a smoky heat component to the final dish. Since beans are high in fiber (and may cause some gas), eat this dish at least a few days before competition. Your body will thank you for the much-needed carbs and protein.

I tablespoon vegetable oil

½ cup chopped yellow onion

I tablespoon diced jalapeño

3 cloves garlic, minced

2 teaspoons smoked paprika

½ teaspoon chili powder

½ teaspoon dried oregano

¼ teaspoon salt

I cup canned fire-roasted tomatoes

I cup long-grain brown rice

I cup low-sodium vegetable broth

I cup water

I can (15.5 oz) kidney beans, drained and rinsed

Warm the vegetable oil in a large pot over medium heat. Add the onion, jalapeño, garlic, paprika, chili powder, oregano, and salt. Cook for 3 to 4 minutes, until the onion is translucent.

Add the tomatoes, rice, broth, water, and beans and bring to a boil. Cover, reduce the heat to low, and simmer for 30 minutes, until all the liquid is absorbed.

Serve immediately or store in a sealed container in the fridge for up to 5 days.

PER SERVING: Calories: 370, Fat: 6g, Sat Fat: 1g, Sodium: 520mg, Carbohydrates: 65g, Dietary Fiber: 10g, Added Sugar: 0g, Protein: 13g, Vitamin D: 0mcg, Calcium: 112mg, Iron: 3mg, Potassium: 437mg

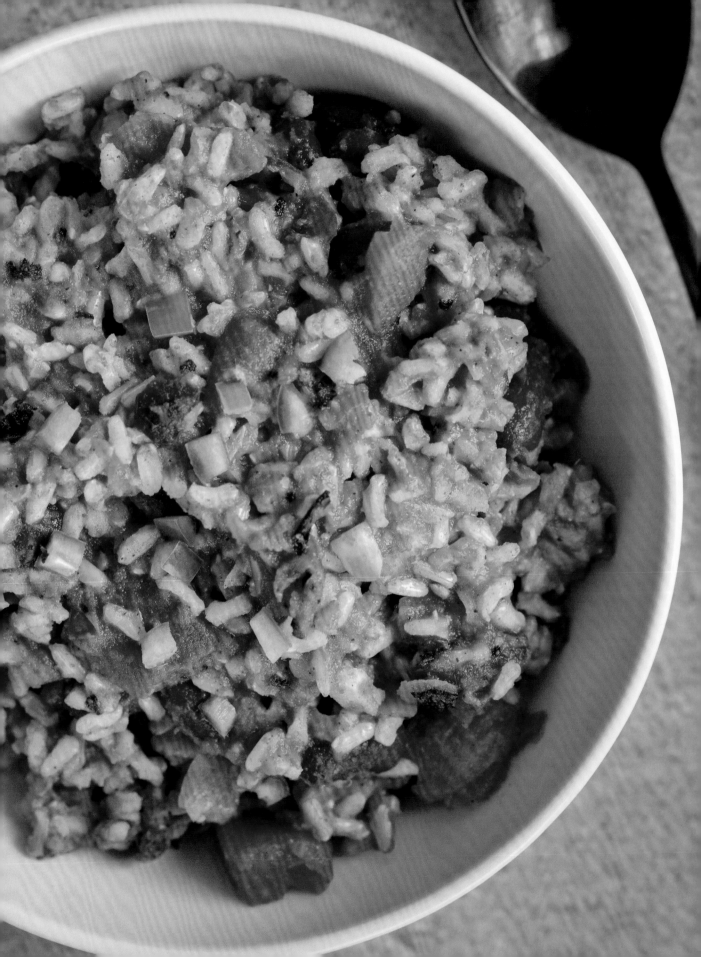

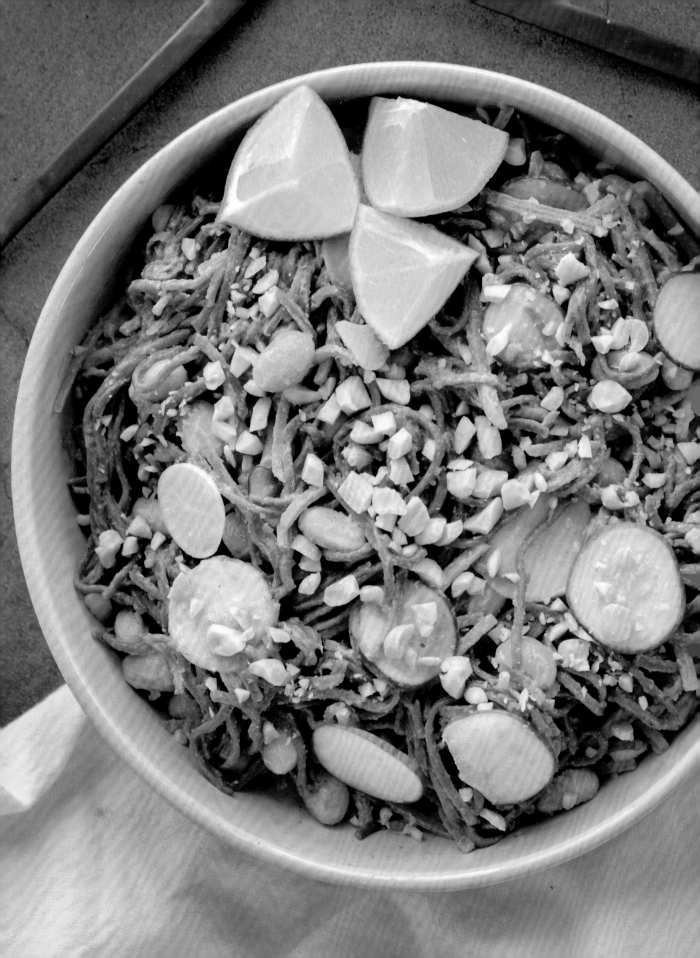

PEANUT SOBA NOODLES

MAKES 4 SERVINGS • PREP TIME: 10 MINUTES / COOK TIME: 10 MINUTES

Soba noodles are a Japanese noodle made from buckwheat flour. Although it has the word "wheat" in the name, buckwheat is actually a gluten-free whole grain that is packed with fiber and protein. If you can't find soba noodles, use whole wheat spaghetti, which also has plenty of fiber and protein. This recipe pairs soba noodles with protein-rich edamame and a peanut sauce, creating a well-balanced dish that can be eaten hot or cold.

FOR THE NOODLES

8 ounces soba noodles or whole wheat spaghetti

¾ cup shelled edamame

½ cup shredded carrots

½ cup sliced radish

FOR THE DRESSING

¼ cup peanut butter

1½ tablespoons sesame oil

2 tablespoons fresh lime juice

1 tablespoon low-sodium soy sauce

1 tablespoon maple syrup

2 tablespoons chopped unsalted roasted peanuts

To make the noodles, bring a large pot of salted water to a boil over high heat. Add the soba noodles and cook according to package directions, usually about 10 minutes. Drain and transfer to a large bowl. Add the edamame, carrots, and radish.

To make the dressing, in a small bowl, whisk together the peanut butter, sesame oil, lime juice, soy sauce, and maple syrup.

Pour the dressing on top of the noodle mixture and toss well. Top with the peanuts and serve immediately or store in a sealed container in the fridge for up to 5 days.

PER SERVING: Calories: 320, Fat: 17g, Sat Fat: 3g, Sodium: 480mg, Carbohydrates: 34g, Dietary Fiber: 3g, Added Sugar: 4g, Protein: 13g, Vitamin D: 0mcg, Calcium: 50mg, Iron: 2mg, Potassium: 370mg

Fun Facts

If you have an intense workout planned for tomorrow morning, choose lower-fiber options for dinner. Instead of whole grains, opt for white rice or white potatoes, and instead of cruciferous vegetables, opt for something starchy, such as carrots, sweet potatoes, or squash.

CAPRESE PASTA SALAD

MAKES 4 SERVINGS • **PREP TIME: 5 MINUTES / COOK TIME: 10 MINUTES**

If you love the flavors of a good caprese salad, you'll really enjoy this pasta salad. Made with farfalle (otherwise known as bow tie) pasta, cherry tomatoes, fresh basil, pesto, and fresh mozzarella, this pasta dish tastes great either warm or cold. The pasta gives you the carb boost you need for heavy training sessions, while the cherry tomatoes are full of antioxidants to fight off inflammation. And as a bonus, this one-pot meal comes together in about 15 minutes.

8 ounces farfalle pasta

2 cups cherry tomatoes, halved

1 cup fresh mozzarella balls or vegan mozzarella

2 tablespoons fresh basil leaves

3 tablespoons pesto

Salt and freshly ground black pepper

Bring a large pot of salted water to a boil over high heat. Add the pasta and cook according to package directions, usually about 10 minutes. Drain the pasta and place it in a large bowl.

Add the tomatoes, mozzarella, basil, and pesto and mix well. Season to taste with salt and black pepper.

Serve immediately as a warm dish or store in a sealed container in the fridge for up to 5 days and serve cold.

PER SERVING: Calories: 350, Fat: 12g, Sat Fat: 4g, Sodium: 450mg, Carbohydrates: 49g, Dietary Fiber: 3g, Added Sugar: 0g, Protein: 14g, Vitamin D: 0mcg, Calcium: 226mg, Iron: 0mg, Potassium: 387mg

Fun Facts

A 3:1 carb-to-protein ratio is ideal for helping muscles recover. Take in 3 grams of carbs for every 1 gram of protein after a workout.

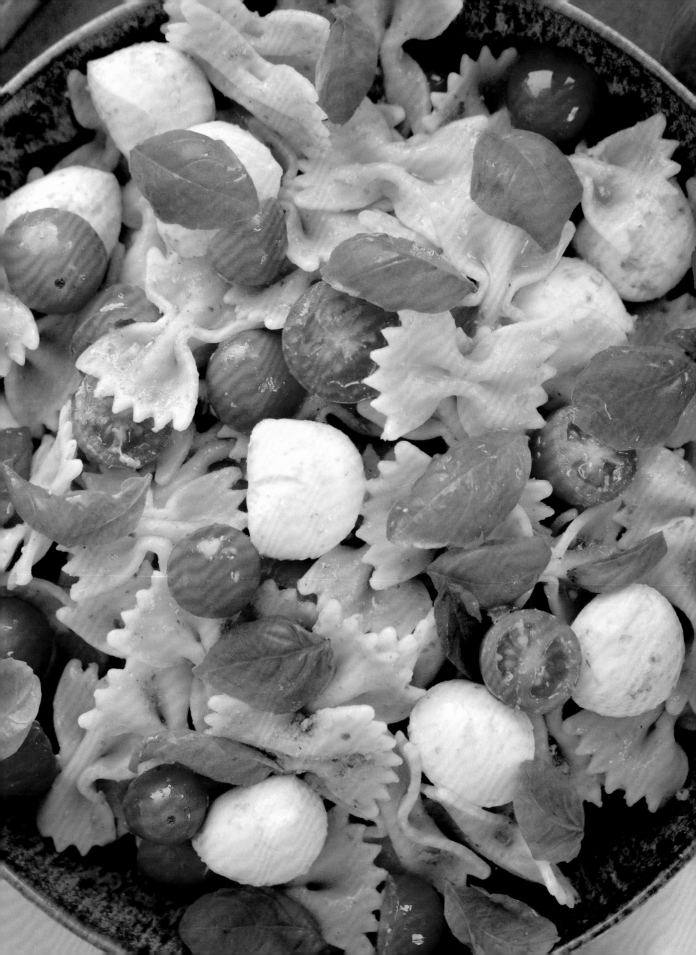

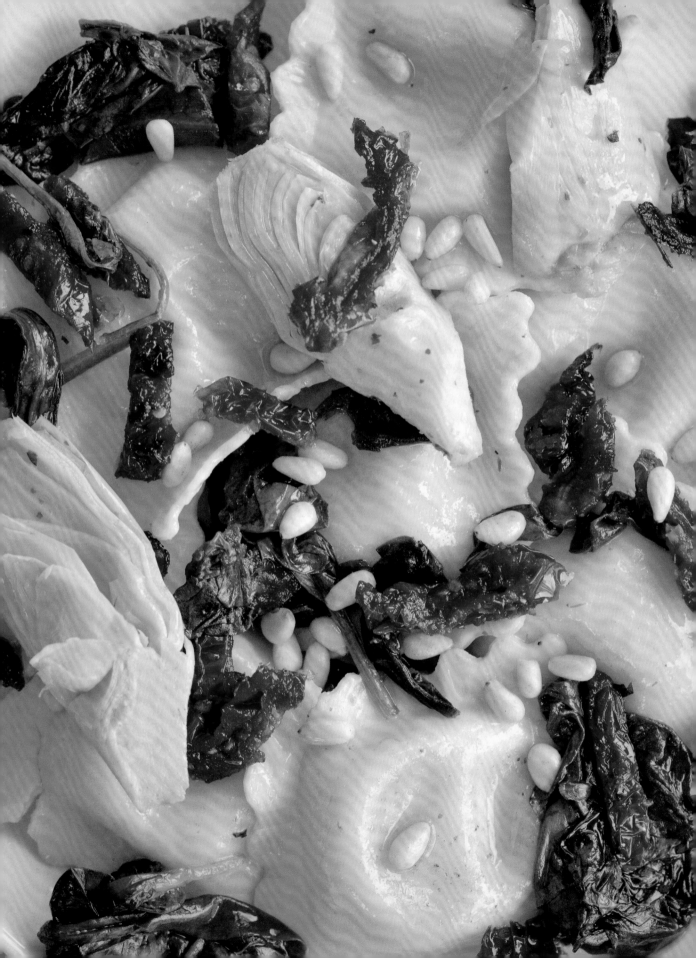

MEDITERRANEAN RAVIOLI BOWL

MAKES 4 SERVINGS • **PREP TIME: 5 MINUTES / COOK TIME: 15 MINUTES**

There's nothing more comforting than stuffed pasta. Ravioli is one of my go-to ingredients because it comes in so many flavors, such as cheese, spinach, butternut squash, and so forth. For this version, I use a cheese ravioli, but feel free to sub in your favorite vegan variety. The only other cooked element is the spinach. Otherwise, the pasta is combined with marinated sun-dried tomatoes and artichokes, both of which come in a jar with olive oil. The sun-dried tomatoes and pine nuts add a wonderful umami flavor to the dish.

- 16 ounces cheese ravioli or vegan ravioli
- 1 tablespoon extra-virgin olive oil
- 4 cups packed spinach
- 2 cups marinated artichokes
- 1 cup marinated sun-dried tomatoes
- Salt and freshly ground black pepper
- ¼ cup unsalted roasted pine nuts

Bring a large pot of water to a boil over high heat. Add the ravioli and cook according to package directions, usually about 10 minutes. Drain and set aside.

In a medium frying pan over medium heat, combine the olive oil, spinach, artichokes, and tomatoes. Cook for 3 to 4 minutes, until the spinach is wilted. Add the cooked ravioli, stir, and remove from the heat. Season to taste with salt and black pepper.

Add the pine nuts and serve immediately. Store leftovers in a sealed container in the fridge for up to 3 days and add pine nuts when ready to serve.

PER SERVING: Calories: 500, Fat: 34g, Sat Fat: 7g, Sodium: 610mg, Carbohydrates: 38g, Dietary Fiber: 6g, Added Sugar: 0g, Protein: 16g, Vitamin D: 1mcg, Calcium: 179mg, Iron: 4mg, Potassium: 740mg

LEMON AND OLIVE OIL GNOCCHI WITH ZUCCHINI RIBBONS

MAKES 4 SERVINGS • **PREP TIME: 5 MINUTES / COOK TIME: 5 MINUTES**

A pasta made from potatoes, gnocchi is a go-to staple for anyone who is carb loading. It cooks quickly and pairs well with practically everything. This superbly simple dish combines gnocchi, zucchini, garlic, olive oil, and lemon juice. It comes together in about 10 minutes, and the ingredients are subtle enough that they won't disrupt the digestive system in the days leading up to an event.

2 pounds gnocchi

1 tablespoon extra-virgin olive oil

3 cloves garlic, minced

2 cups zucchini ribbons

2 tablespoons fresh lemon juice

¼ teaspoon salt

Pepper to taste

Bring a large pot of water to a boil over high heat. Add the gnocchi and cook according to package directions, usually about 2 minutes. Drain and set aside.

Meanwhile, in a sauté pan over medium heat, cook the olive oil and garlic for 1 to 2 minutes, until the garlic begins to brown.

Add the cooked gnocchi, zucchini, lemon juice, salt, and pepper and cook for 2 minutes longer, until warmed through.

Serve immediately or store in a sealed container in the fridge for up to 3 days.

PER SERVING: Calories: 350, Fat: 18g, Sat Fat: 9g, Sodium: 810mg, Carbohydrates: 42g, Dietary Fiber: 1g, Added Sugar: 0g, Protein: 6g, Vitamin D: 0mcg, Calcium: 62mg, Iron: 2mg, Potassium: 483mg

Tip: Use a vegetable peeler to shave zucchini into "ribbons."

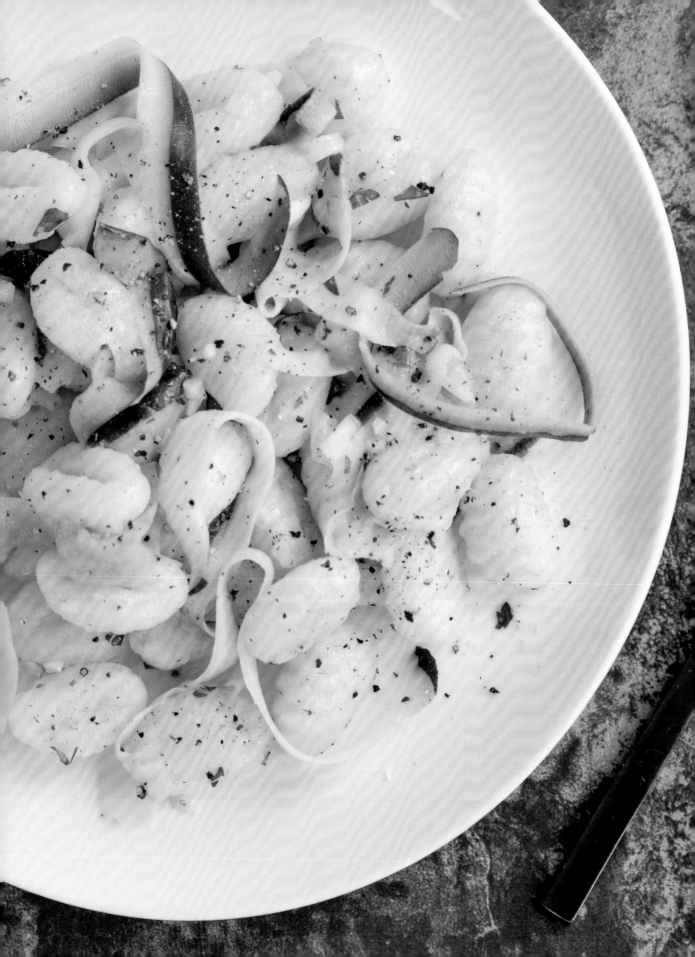

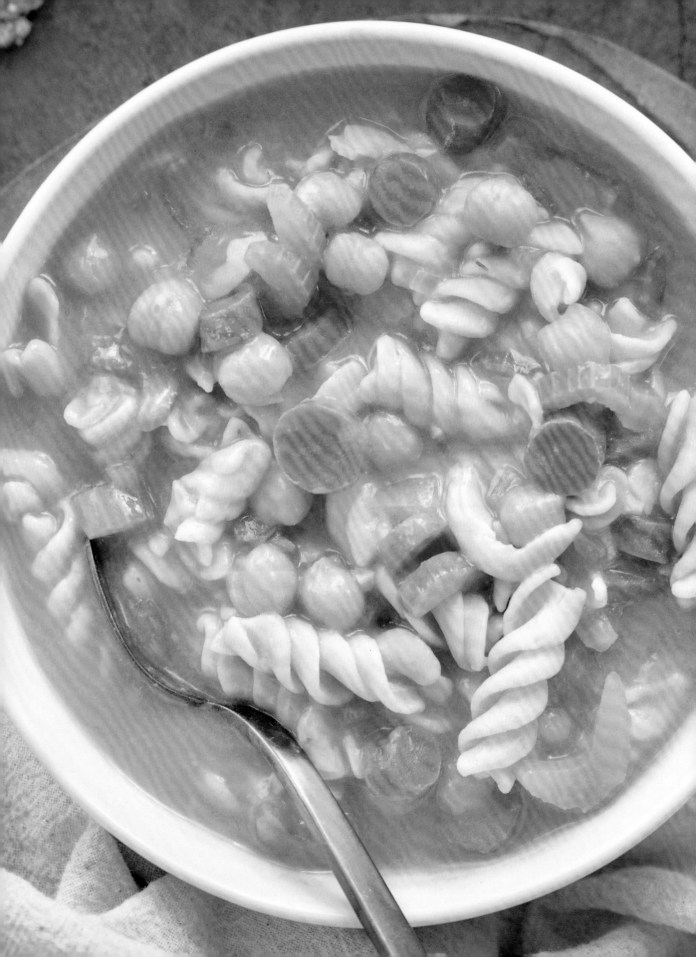

CHICKPEA NOODLE SOUP

MAKES 4 SERVINGS • PREP TIME: 10 MINUTES / COOK TIME: 30 MINUTES

This soup is a vegan play on one of the most comforting soups around—chicken noodle soup. Rather than using chicken and chicken broth, it features chickpeas and vegetable broth. Big chunks of celery, carrot, and onion are simmered in a salty broth with bean-based fusilli pasta. Of course, you can use whatever type of pasta you have on hand, but I recommend those made from chickpeas, lentils, or other beans for an added protein boost.

I tablespoon extra-virgin olive oil

I cup sliced carrot

I cup sliced celery

½ cup diced white onion

2 cloves garlic, minced

½ teaspoon salt

¼ teaspoon dried thyme

6 ounces bean-based fusilli pasta

7 cups low-sodium vegetable broth

I can (15.5 oz) chickpeas, drained and rinsed

Warm the olive oil in a large stockpot over medium heat. Add the carrot, celery, onion, garlic, salt, and thyme. Stir and cook for 4 to 5 minutes, until the onion is translucent.

Add the pasta and broth and bring to a boil. Cook for 7 to 8 minutes, until the pasta is tender. Add the chickpeas, reduce the heat to low, and simmer, uncovered, for 15 minutes, until the flavors meld.

Serve immediately or store in a sealed container in the fridge for up to 5 days or in the freezer for up to 3 months. Defrost in a large stockpot over medium heat and serve hot.

PER SERVING: Calories: 380, Fat: 8g, Sat Fat: 0.5g, Sodium: 800mg, Carbohydrates: 63g, Dietary Fiber: 9g, Added Sugar: 3g, Protein: 17g, Vitamin D: 0mcg, Calcium: 110mg, Iron: 4mg, Potassium: 604mg

Vegan Tip: Save the chickpea liquid, called "aquafaba," which can be used as an egg replacer in many baked dishes.

SUMMER VEGGIE FARRO RISOTTO

MAKES 4 SERVINGS • PREP TIME: 5 MINUTES / COOK TIME: 30 MINUTES

A good risotto takes a lot of time and energy to make, and it's usually loaded with butter and cheese. This version is different. You start with whole grain quick-cooking farro, which eliminates much of the cooking time but still absorbs the liquid. Then add flavorful summer veggies, such as tomatoes and corn, and top it off with cheese or nutritional yeast. It's the perfect carb-rich dish to make in a big batch for a week of heavy training.

1 tablespoon extra-virgin olive oil

1 cup cherry tomatoes, halved

1 cup unsalted corn kernels

⅓ cup chopped fresh chives

2 cloves garlic, minced

¼ teaspoon salt

1½ cups quick-cooking farro

½ cup dry white wine

3 cups low-sodium vegetable broth

½ cup vegetarian parmesan cheese (see tip)

Vegan Tip: Sub ¼ cup of nutritional yeast for the parmesan cheese. Add more if desired.

In a large pot over medium heat, combine the olive oil, tomatoes, corn, chives, garlic, and salt. Cook for 3 to 5 minutes, until the vegetables start to brown.

Add the farro and stir. Cook for 1 to 2 minutes, until all the ingredients are coated in oil. Add the white wine and let the liquid absorb (this happens quickly). Add 1 cup of broth, reduce the heat to low, and simmer, uncovered, for 5 minutes, until the broth is almost absorbed.

Add another 1 cup of broth. Cook, stirring, for 5 minutes, until the broth is absorbed. Add the remaining 1 cup of broth and cook, stirring, for 10 minutes, until most of the broth is absorbed.

Remove the farro from the heat and add the cheese, stirring until combined.

Serve immediately or store in a sealed container in the fridge for up to 5 days or in the freezer for up to 3 months. When ready to eat, place it in a pot with ¼ cup of vegetable broth and warm until defrosted.

PER SERVING: Calories: 460, Fat: 12g, Sat Fat: 4.5g, Sodium: 500mg, Carbohydrates: 64g, Dietary Fiber: 9g, Added Sugar: 1g, Protein: 19g, Vitamin D: 0mcg, Calcium: 381mg, Iron: 2mg, Potassium: 511mg

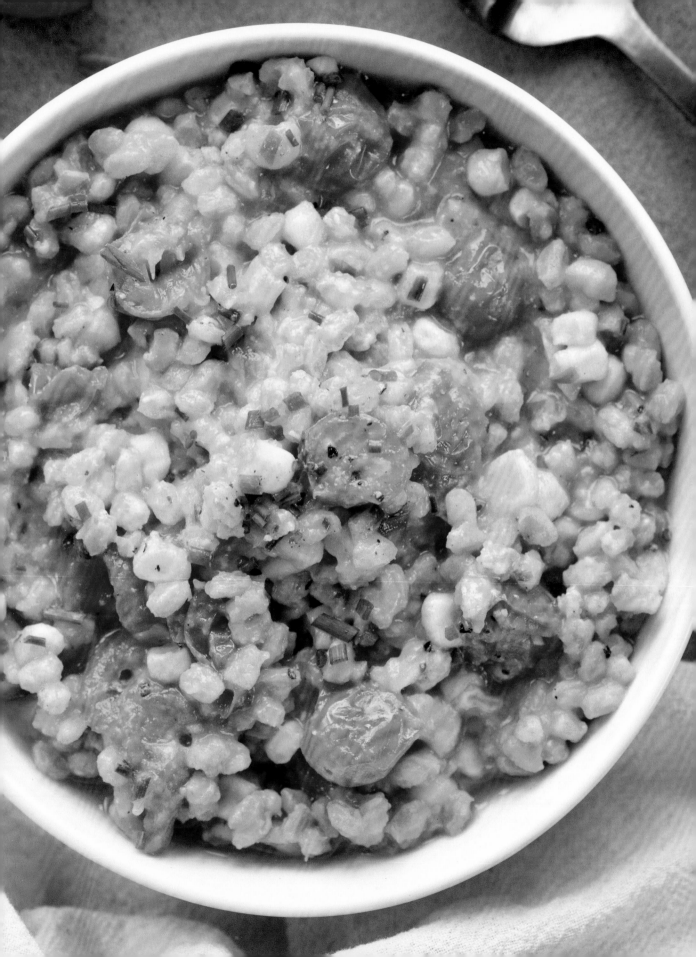

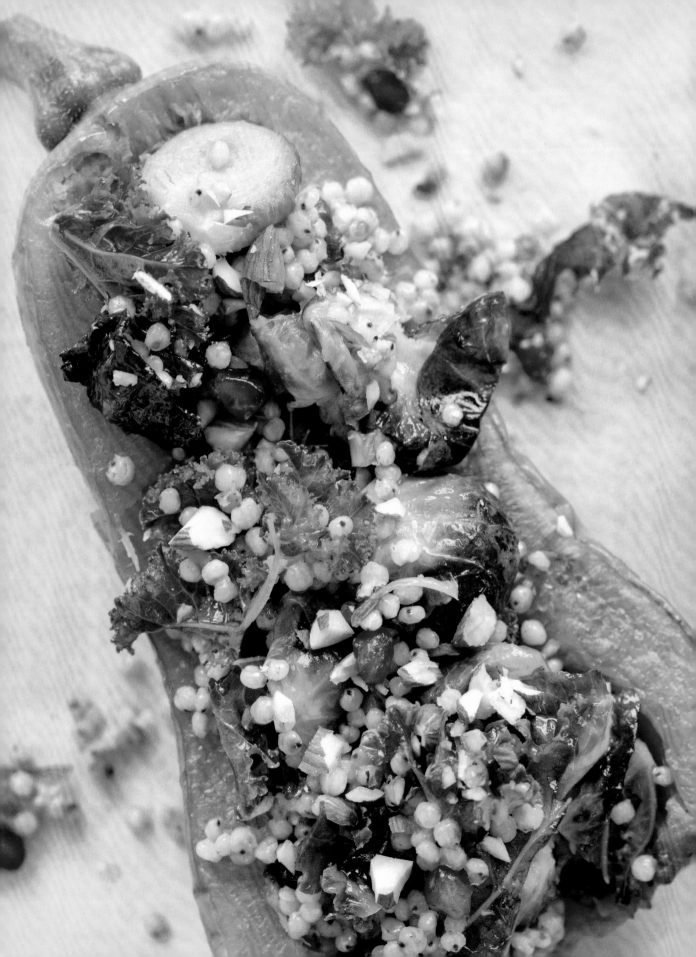

STUFFED BUTTERNUT SQUASH WITH SORGHUM

MAKES 4 SERVINGS • PREP TIME: 5 MINUTES / COOK TIME: 1 HOUR

Sorghum is a powerhouse grain that isn't used nearly enough. It has protein, B vitamins, magnesium, and potassium. A ½-cup serving (uncooked) yields around 1¾ cups of cooked sorghum with 10 grams of plant-based protein, 69 grams of carbohydrates, and 6 grams of dietary fiber.

FOR THE SQUASH

1 pound brussels sprouts, halved

2 tablespoons extra-virgin olive oil

2 butternut squash, halved lengthwise and seeded

1 cup dried sorghum

2 cups chopped stemmed kale

½ cup pomegranate seeds

¼ teaspoon salt

FOR THE DRESSING

¼ cup extra-virgin olive oil

2 tablespoons apple cider vinegar

1 tablespoon Dijon mustard

1 tablespoon honey or maple syrup

¼ teaspoon salt

Preheat the oven to 400°F. Line a baking sheet with parchment paper.

To make the squash, in a large bowl, toss the sprouts with 1 tablespoon of olive oil and set aside. Drizzle the remaining 1 tablespoon of olive oil over the flesh of the squash. Place it facedown on the prepared baking sheet. Bake for 20 minutes. Add the sprouts to the baking sheet and cook for 20 minutes longer, until the edges of the squash are golden brown and the sprouts are brown around the edges.

Meanwhile, cook the sorghum according to package directions, usually about 1 hour.

Transfer the cooked sorghum to a large bowl. Add the roasted sprouts, kale, pomegranate seeds, and salt and stir.

To make the dressing, in a small bowl, whisk together the olive oil, vinegar, mustard, honey, and salt.

Pour the dressing over the sorghum mixture and mix well. Spoon the sorghum mixture onto the cooked squash halves and eat directly out of the skin. Do not eat the skin—it's very chewy.

Serve immediately or store in a sealed container in the fridge for up to 5 days.

PER SERVING: Calories: 480, Fat: 22g, Sat Fat: 3g, Sodium: 390mg, Carbohydrates: 67g, Dietary Fiber: 16g, Added Sugar: 4g, Protein: 10g, Vitamin D: 0mcg, Calcium: 108mg, Iron: 5mg, Potassium: 1,195mg

ACKNOWLEDGMENTS

Many hardworking and passionate people helped me bring this book to life. I'm honored to know all of you, and please let me share my gratitude with: Sara Gilligan, my literary agent, who turned my idea into a reality. This book would still be buzzing around my head if it weren't for you. Claire Yee and John Foster, my editors, and the entire Weldon Owen team for keeping me organized and transforming my hours of labor into a book that I'm proud to share with the world. I wouldn't have been able to do this without your expertise and patience. Georgina Keriby-Smith, for your help with all the nutrition analysis. Your attention to detail is unmatched. Bill Paetzke, my husband, who tasted every recipe and kept the baby out of my hair while I finished this project. Thanks for being supportive and encouraging and for loving plants as much as I do.

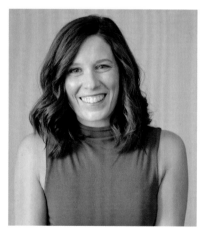

ABOUT THE AUTHOR

Natalie Rizzo, MS, RD is a NYC-based media dietitian, food and nutrition writer, national spokesperson, and owner of Greenletes®, a successful plant-based sports nutrition blog and podcast. Natalie has bylines in many national publications, such as NBC News, SHAPE, *Runner's World*, *Bicycling*, *Diabetic Living*, and *Prevention*. In her work as a nutrition spokesperson, she frequently appears in television segments and is quoted as the nutrition expert in top-tier national publications. Natalie is passionate about simplifying complicated sports nutrition information for everyday athletes, and she's dedicated to teaching them how to eat more plants. She's been a vegetarian for over a decade and a runner for almost as long. She resides in New York City with her husband and son. Find her on Instagram @greenletes, visit her website at greenletes.com, and listen to the Greenletes Podcast.

TABLE OF EQUIVALENTS

The exact equivalents in the following tables have been rounded for convenience.

LIQUID AND DRY MEASUREMENTS

U.S.	METRIC
¼ teaspoon	1.25 milliliters
½ teaspoon	2.5 milliliters
I teaspoon	5 milliliters
I tablespoon (3 teaspoons)	15 milliliters
I fluid ounce	30 milliliters
¼ cup	60 milliliters
⅓ cup	80 milliliters
I cup	235 milliliters
I pint (2 cups)	480 milliliters
I quart (4 cups, 32 fluid ounces)	950 milliliters
I gallon (4 quarts)	3.8 liters
I ounce (by weight)	28 grams
I pound	454 grams
2.2 pounds	I kilogram

LENGTH MEASURES

U.S.	METRIC
⅛ inch	6 millimeters
½ inch	12 millimeters
I inch	2.5 centimeters

OVEN TEMPERATURES

FAHRENHEIT	CELSIUS	GAS
250°	120°	½
275°	140°	I
300°	150°	2
325°	160°	3
350°	180°	4
375°	190°	5
400°	200°	6
425°	220°	7
450°	230°	8
475°	240°	9
500°	260°	10

INDEX

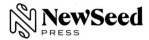

an imprint of Insight Editions
P.O. Box 3088
San Rafael, CA 94912
www.weldonowen.com

CEO Raoul Goff
VP Publisher Roger Shaw
Editorial Director Katie Killebrew
Senior Editor John Foster
Editor Claire Yee
Editorial Assistant: Kayla Belser-Vernon
VP Creative Chrissy Kwasnik
Designers Rita Sowins and Amy DeGrote
VP Manufacturing Alix Nicholaeff
Production Manager Joshua Smith
Sr Production Manager, Subsidiary Rights Lina s Palma-Temena

New Seed Press would also like to thank Jessica Easto for copyediting, Mary J. Cassells
for proofreading, and Timothy Griffin for indexing.

Text © 2023 by Natalie Rizzo, MS, RD
Food photography © 2023 by Natalie Rizzo, MS, RD

All rights reserved. No part of this book may be reproduced in any form without written
permission from the publisher.

ISBN: 978-1-68188-858-3

Manufactured in 2023 by Insight Editions
10 9 8 7 6 5 4 3 2 1

Disclaimer: The information in this book is provided as a resource for inspiration and nutrition
education. It is not prescriptive, but may be used to complement the care of a qualified health
professional. Author and Publisher expressly disclaim any responsibility for any adverse effects
from the use or application of the information contained in this book. Neither the Publisher nor
Author shall be liable for any losses suffered by any reader of this book.

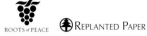

Insight Editions, in association with Roots of Peace, will plant two trees for each tree used in the
manufacturing of this book. Roots of Peace is an internationally renowned humanitarian organiza-
tion dedicated to eradicating land mines worldwide and converting war-torn lands into productive
farms and wildlife habitats. Roots of Peace will plant two million fruit and nut trees in Afghanistan
and provide farmers there with the skills and support necessary for sustainable land use.